His was a very different professional world. His arrogant orders were obeyed instantly and without question. Before the arrival of antibiotics and vaccines — during the dark ages of infectious diseases, malnutrition and ignorance — there is no doubt that his dogmatic insistence on specific treatments and procedures saved thousands of lives. Such positive results brought increasing international acclaim to the hospital. His students spread across Canada to become chiefs of paediatrics at other teaching hospitals. He himself did not receive the international recognition that his leadership won for his hospital.

Those blessed with great skills are often cursed with great defects. Alan Brown was no exception. He was a man with a purpose so big that he built an ego to match it. He always thought his decisions were right and he allowed no one to stand in his way.

Chapter 1

The Locked Door

JANUARY 1949

The blizzard that had begun the night before continued all morning. The snow was thick and heavy, the footing precarious. The Class of '50 was larger than usual. Close to 200 medical students were taking instruction at several teaching hospitals in the city and in the University of Toronto. At a brisk walk in good weather the usual ten minutes between classes gave barely enough time to reach the amphitheatre in the old Sick Children's Hospital on College Street where Alan Brown held his lectures. He had given fair warning that late arrivals would be locked out. He did not tolerate interruptions during his lectures. Sometimes students left their preceding class or clinic early to be on time. On the day of the blizzard, at ten minutes past the hour, Alan Brown locked the door. Delayed by the winter storm, more than half the class arrived late and missed the lecture. Several weeks later, Alan Brown himself was late and the class retaliated by locking the door on him. The fat was in the fire. Alan Brown was not amused and did not lecture that day. Some of today's most distinguished older members of the medical profession, including those who were students in that class, contradict one another in their recollections of what happened. Listen to their accounts:

Alan Brown's successor
He was the Professor . . . a very busy man, always punctual. A case can

be made for both sides. He didn't like having his class interrupted by late arrivals and his students didn't like being treated as children. When they locked him out that day he told the Dean of Medicine (Joe McFarlane) that he wouldn't continue his classes until he got an apology. He got it — he didn't have to wait very long. (Dr. A. Lawrence Chute, Dean of the Faculty of Medicine, University of Toronto. Retired.)

Student, Class of '39
He was a superb lecturer but a very unpleasant character. His lectures were held in the old amphitheatre that had steeply-raked seats. If you were late, it was hard to sneak in and up the stairs to the back rows. He didn't lock the door, not when I was there. Sometimes a late student would try to creep in and climb up to the back. Alan Brown would stop his lecture, point his finger and say, "Get out of this room; you are wasting precious minutes. There are one hundred and forty in this class and you've wasted two minutes of their time, that's two hundred and eighty minutes. You're a thief." He did have a point. (Dr. Robert MacMillan, emeritus professor, University of Toronto)

One of Alan Brown's junior staff
I was at the hospital at that time. The class was largely made up of RCAF[1]* and army guys — a lot of them had been POWs.[2] Some of us had pointed out to Alan that they deserved a certain amount of respect, that this gang was a different kettle of fish. His habit was to lock the door when he came into the room so that he wouldn't be disturbed during the course of his lecture. The blizzard delayed the class. They had to boot it across Queen's Park or up from St. Mike's to get to Sick Kids. There was one guy who'd lost his foot in a 'plane crash and then was taken prisoner of war.[3] He couldn't make it across the park in very good time through all the snow. He and many others were late. Alan had locked the door as usual and he lectured to about one third of the class. A couple of weeks later he was late. The class locked the door. There was hell to pay. He was absolutely furious. He ranted and he raved. I remember listening to him. He demanded an apology. I think the guys were justifiably angry about the whole thing but realized that there wasn't any future in keeping the old boy in a state of constant angina. So the class president ulti-

---

* For all numbers or letter references please see Notes section at back of book.

mately did apologize. He accepted the apology and went back to giving his lectures. It was two or three weeks before the whole thing simmered down. Alan never locked the door again. He'd learned a lesson, but oh, it was a tough lesson. (Dr. J.A. Peter Turner, FRCPC)

Student, Class of '50
Our class was larger than usual, nearly all ex-service returning from overseas. We were used to heavy responsibilities and we were older than the usual med student. Many of us had been prisoners of war and Scrimgeour had been shot down, captured and lost a leg. For these reasons we were a unique group back on civvy street, many of us still in uniform. I'd heard enough about Dr. Alan Brown's classes to know what to expect. But some of the other chaps would mutter, "Who is this arrogant bastard? We're not just out of prep school." We had all returned with a big purpose, and minor things like Alan Brown's teaching tactics didn't bother us much. He expected his whole class to be there seated with pencils poised and ready to write when he arrived. We'd stand up when he came in and after his "Sit down please" he'd begin to lecture. The door was locked once he was in. That day we were all there and we kept looking at our watches. Everybody was champing at the bit. "Where is the professor? He's late." Then someone said, "Lock him out." There was a good deal of agreement to the idea. I think Sudsy Sutherland may have been the one who locked the door. Then we waited and waited, five or six minutes at the most. At last we heard footsteps approaching. The door handle turned, not once or twice but three times. Then the footsteps retreated. Into the dead silence someone said, "Oh! Oh!." We thought he'd treat it as a joke. Someone unlocked the door and shortly after Phil Rance[4] came in and announced, "I've a message from Dr. Brown. He's pretty upset and has asked me to tell you at the next class there will be a written test on the subject matter that he was going to lecture on today." I thought that was pretty smart and we deserved it. But now, looking back, it was a juvenile thing to do — on both sides. (Dr. Colin S. Ross, lately Vice-President and Medical Director of Munich Reinsurance Company of Canada)

Alan Brown's clinic nurse
As for that class locking him out, he couldn't treat it as a joke. He dropped everything for the sake of coming and giving those lectures. I never knew

him to be late. Obviously one day he was, and the students took advantage of him. No matter what happened he was always there for that class. There was so little time allotted to paediatrics in the general curriculum. He wasn't trying to make them specialists. He just wanted them to know enough to recognize and treat everyday things and to know when to call in somebody else. Nothing was allowed to interfere with his teaching — neither his hospital responsibilities nor his private practice. (Margaret D. Neilson, RN)

Student, Class of '50
Bill Hogg was a big, tall, gangly fellow with extra joints all over the place and a great big smile. Can't remember who suggested it but it was Bill who snapped the lock. I was pretty surprised and thought, Holy Joe! Because I didn't think he would treat it as a joke. Then, I remember the door handle turning — rattle, rattle, rattle. We could see a silhouette through the frosted glass panel. Then it was gone. Alan Bruce-Robertson quietly walked over and unlocked the door. When Phil Rance came in with that long thin nose of his, I thought it meant trouble: "Dr. Brown is not going to lecture to this group again till he gets a written apology." The story made the rounds. Harold Reichert,[5] a good teacher and a big bluff guy, was in the TGH with a heart attack. When he heard about it he laughed so hard he fell out of bed. Ken Mackenzie[6] had a wonderful sense of humour and the next day when he came to lecture to us, he scratched his head and he could hardly speak he was laughing so hard. "You certainly stir things up when you get started, don't you?" Those guys liked to see Alan Brown discomfited. They thought he was a pompous ass. But he never did lock the door! He said he would, but even on that stormy day when we were all late he never did it. The only time I can remember it being locked was the day we locked him out. Allman[7] was the class president that year and a couple of days later while we were waiting for a lecture in the TGH, I remember him reading aloud the letter he was going to deliver to Alan Brown. "Now look, you guys. This is what I've been told we have to do. You're all here so I want to read you this thing and if you have any objections, sing out." We all heehawed and booed and since it didn't say very much, we let it go. When we finally got back on track and Alan Brown returned to lecture, there was no reference made to the episode — none. Probably too much

has been made of the incident. (Dr. Walter F. Prendergast, Physician to the T. Eaton Company)

Student, Class of '50, Alan Brown's godson
We could understand that he did not want anyone coming in the front door by the podium but we didn't understand why we couldn't slip in quietly by the side door which was high up towards the back. He had his resident go up and lock that door as well. Well, one day he was late and someone locked the door. When he arrived with a resident in tow, there was a bit of rattling as the handle turned and I guess it was the chief resident[8] who called out, "It's Dr. Brown. Let him in." Then we heard them retreating. I unlocked the door. Five or ten minutes later a resident, I think it was Rance, came all the way around and up to enter the back door. We hadn't locked it. "Dr. Brown is not very pleased and he demands an apology." Reg Allman who was our class president concocted it. We agreed it sounded sufficiently like an apology and Uncle Alan accepted it. We were back in class the next week, almost as though nothing had ever happened. I don't remember an exam but it's the sort of thing he would do. He was the only professor in the whole faculty who insisted on locking his door. He was unrealistic, acting as though there was no other life, no other lectures but his. If he'd had any sense of humour he'd have called through the door, "Well, you got me, now let me in, let's get on with it." Some of us were still chuckling when Rance appeared. (Dr. Alan Bruce-Robertson, Research Associate, University of Toronto)

Alan Brown's Chief Resident 1949-50
That day Dr. Brown and I carried on our usual morning routine in the hospital, then walked to the lecture theatre. We tried the door and rattled the knob. It was locked and no one came to unlock it for him. He became very angry at their lack of respect and barked at me, "Tell that class I'll not lecture again until I receive an apology." Once the apology was given the episode was over — it was no big deal — but he continued to lock the door against latecomers. (Dr. Donald R. Clark, Paediatrician, Peterborough)

One of Alan Brown's residents
There was a famous incident when I was a resident. He was a stickler

for time. "My lectures start at twelve o'clock, everybody's in at twelve o'clock and the door is locked." There was a reason for locking the front door because you had to cross right in front of him as he was lecturing to the students — very disruptive. The upper side door was always open but if you crept in that way a few minutes or even seconds late, then you could count on being ridiculed throughout that entire period. One day he was late. His students locked him out. There was hell to pay. He threatened to fail every single member of the class so they wouldn't get their degrees. He demanded a formal apology. He got it, and he should have got it. (Dr. Robert Farber, Paediatrician, HSC)

One of Alan Brown's senior colleagues
I don't think his reaction was childish. They had no right to lock him out. He was not like the heads of hospitals now that just deal with finance and administration. He was responsible for running the whole hospital in addition to his medical and teaching duties plus a large private practice. If a bunch of students locked him out he would be furious. It was HIS hospital and HE called the shots. (Dr. Nelles Silverthorne, Honorary Consultant HSC)

The latest published version
Dr. Brown . . . arrived ten minutes past the hour to find the lecture room door . . . locked. A few minutes later he entered by a small, side door at the rear of the theatre to find the ex-servicemen laughing and thoroughly enjoying their joke. With great glee they informed him that he was late. The professor promptly turned on his heel, left the classroom and headed for his office. He refused to teach that . . . class again until he received a formal apology. Four scheduled lecture periods passed untaught, . . . finally the apology was forthcoming and normal teaching resumed.[9]

"The Locked Door" story sifted through the hospital and out into the medical community. Its various versions were often contradictory. After forty years, even those who took part in the episode remember it differently. Their shaky memories illustrate the strong positive and negative reactions that Alan Brown attracted throughout his professional life. Who was right and who was wrong? Was Alan Brown in the habit of locking the door? Or did he merely warn that he would? No one will ever know the full story of The Locked Door. Controversy churned around the incident and blew it out of proportion. It became famous, one of many examples of a reputation for eccentricity that grew and clung to Alan Brown throughout his long tenure as the University's professor of paediatrics and The Hospital for Sick Children's physician-in-chief. "He was a figure of legend and controversy, a mixture of vanity and medical excellence. He was magnanimous yet petty, and failed to appreciate the intended humour of the locked door."[10] A man less jealous of his position and less intense about the importance of his teaching would have joined in the joke. Alan Brown could not. He thought his classes too important to be treated lightly. A dedicated teacher, he expected his students to take his classes seriously.

ACADEMY OF MEDICINE, TORONTO
13 QUEEN'S PARK

The Academy of Medicine, Toronto, is desirous of having on file biographical notes on all Fellows, past and present. You are requested to detach and fill in this form at your earliest convenience and return to the Honorary Secretary.

Name *Alan Brown* Father *George W Brown*
Birth (Date) *1867* Mother's Maiden Name *Gavina Gowans*
Place *Toronto* Religion *United Church*
University and Honorary Degrees and dates *M.D. 1909 ; F.R.C.P.(L.S) Lond. 1940*

Post-Graduate Work *New York, Berlin, Hopitae, Vienna; Austria, Denmark, London*

Practice *Pediatrics*

Military Service *none*

Married (date, place, and wife's name) *Jan 1914 — Constance Hills*

Children (names) *Barbara, Nancy, Chauncer de Vecise J (deceased) 1918-19, Member of Council 1919-20.*

Hospital Appointments Physician-in-Chief, Hospital for Sick Children, Toronto.
Consulting Physician to Riverdale Isolation Hospital, Toronto.
" Women's College Hospital,
Consulting Paediatrician to Newborn Clinic, Toronto General Hospital, Toronto.
" " Infants' Home, Toronto
" " Local, Provincial and Dominion Departments of Health.

University Appointments
Professor of Paediatrics, University of Toronto.

Contributions to Medical Science
In Collaboration with F.F. Tisdall & R.S. M'Bride developed infant foods known to public.

Contributions to Medical Literature (List may be attached)
See attached list.

Additional Information
Author of "The Normal Child, Its Care and Feeding", 3rd Ed.
Senior Author - with F.F.Tisdall - "Common Procedures in the Practice of Paediatrics". 3rd Ed.
Corresponding member of the British Paediatric Society.
Honorary member of the North Pacific Coast Pediatric Society
" " " " Dallas, Texas, Clinical Society
Fellow of the American College of Physicians
" " " American Academy of Pediatrics
Past President, Canadian Society for the Study of Diseases of Children

Date *February 24, 1943* Signed *Alan Brown*
Address *51 Oriole Rd.*

(ATTACH BLANK SHEET, IF MORE SPACE REQUIRED)

Toronto Academy of Medicine questionnaire, 1943

— Chapter 2 —
Ahead of His Time

AUTHORITIES differ over the year of Alan Brown's birth. The United States' Library of Congress in its *National Union Catalogue of Books* states 1885 in all its entries for his publications. The Homewood Medical Centre in Guelph, Ontario, records 1886, and Alan Brown himself writes 1887 in his reply to a 1943 Toronto Academy of Medicine questionnaire. The year may be in doubt but the day is not. He was born prematurely on the twenty-seventh of September in an era when premature babies suffered a very high mortality rate. He told Howard McGarry, his chief resident in 1934, that he was a sickly child and that his parents had a hard time raising him. Fortunately he lived to save the lives of thousands of infants and children. To have survived prematurity at that time was no doubt partly due to his mother's two-year stint in medical school.

Alan passed his early childhood in Clinton, Ontario, where his two brothers Clinton and Donald and his sister Margery were born. They grew up during the height of the Victorian era when appearance was valued more than substance. Piano legs hid behind skirts, women's hems swept the floor and the bustle, in defiance of the prescribed code of female modesty, was the universal fashion. One outraged father ordered his daughter, "You are not to wear that dress again. I saw you on Main Street this afternoon; you were wearing a hump and it was waggling!"[1]

Horse-drawn carriages and unpaved streets forced pedestrians to pick their way cautiously through the mud and manure of the city's main streets, keeping an eye out for streetcars drawn by teams of easily distracted and unpredictable horses. It was not an uncommon sight to see a runaway team careening down the street, its trolley lurching from side to side and its terrified passengers hanging on, silently praying or loudly cursing.

It was a conspicuously devout age. Religious routines, predominantly Protestant, were followed to the letter. Obligatory Sunday church attendance was at the same time treated as a social occasion where stylish clothes were the order of the day. The pursuit of impressing one's neighbours was relentless. Conformity and discipline were the paramount features of social behaviour throughout Ontario. Children were to be seen and not heard. Many attended one-room schoolhouses where sometimes their teachers knew little more than they did. Childhood diseases were rampant and the death rate was high. Life expectancy at birth was under fifty years. Proper sanitation was rudimentary or non-existent and indoor plumbing was the exception rather than the rule. Privies at the bottom of the garden were common. Lem Pott's helpful and hilarious advice on privy building would have shocked but delighted many, even in Victorian Canada. Certainly forty years later it provoked eruptions of helpless laughter as Alan and his wife followed its illustrated directions.[2]

Late nineteenth century immigrants from "the mother country" had been attracted by crown land grants and the relative political and social stability Canada offered. The country had put behind it earlier wars and rebellions. The Americans had been defeated in their attempt to annex Canada by invasion in the War of 1812; William Lyon Mackenzie's rebellion of the 1830s and Louis Riel's in the 1870s were history.

In 1867 the Confederation of Canada was painfully negotiated at an historic meeting in Charlottetown where representatives from Nova Scotia, New Brunswick, Upper and Lower Canada rather reluctantly decided to unite, more for protection than for shared interests. These so-called Fathers of Confederation had become nervous when the American Civil War ended in 1865. They feared the United States might again focus its territorial ambitions on its northern neighbour just as it had in the War of 1812. Thus Canada backed into nationhood; an inauspicious beginning but typical of the many compromises this unwieldy country has come to accept.

The disparate citizens of the new nation were fascinated by the novelty of electing a truly national government. Politics took precedence over religion as topics for dispute in and out of the home. The achievements of Canada's first Prime Minister, Sir John A. Macdonald, were as widely discussed as his favourite vice, a startling capacity for Scotch whisky. At debates in the Commons the whisky was discreetly replaced by clear gin in a tumbler. His vision of uniting Canada from sea to sea by a transcontinental railway became a reality when Donald Smith (later created Baron Strathcona and Mount Royal) drove the last spike into place in 1885. At the time of Alan Brown's birth one or two years later, Prince Edward Island, Manitoba and British Columbia had also joined the Confederation of Canada.

When they were very young, Alan's parents, George Brown and Gavina Gowans, and their families had immigrated to Canada from Scotland. They were married in the early 1880s after Gavina's second year at the Toronto Women's Medical College, where many of the female students were taught until 1906 when the University of Toronto at last admitted them. Perhaps too hastily, Gavina chose marriage and a family over medicine. As the years passed her by she became increasingly bitter and her frequent caustic remarks suggest that she regretted her decision to abandon medical training. There is no doubt that she influenced her eldest son to think of medicine as a career.

Gavina Gowans Brown was a difficult woman to love, judging by the way all her grown children avoided her. At Alan's graduation in 1909 from the University of Toronto Medical School (with the Silver Medal) she was venomous. "He would have won the Gold if he hadn't been taking out that Hobbs girl." The remark made the rounds and did not endear her to her future daughter-in-law who never spoke to her again. In fact, Alan's father and mother were not even invited to their wedding four years later and Alan quietly dropped his middle name, Gowans, from his published work. Only on his early papers is his mother's maiden name included as part of his own.

Perhaps she was a little unbalanced by her unsatisfied dreams and disappointments in life. There was also evidence of mental instability in her family. One of her sisters suffered from a permanent "nervous breakdown". Alan had warned his Aunt Susan that she was working too hard and should slow down. Susan lived with her sister Grace Gowans, a graduate nurse, who devoted the rest of her life to caring for her. Alan was very fond of his mother's sisters and often dropped in for tea at their duplex on Dupont Street at Avenue Road and later to their house on

Woodlawn Avenue. They always made a big fuss over their nephew and Alan basked in the warmth of their attentions. A fourth sister, Aunt Annie, became a missionary in China, returning home for holidays at irregular intervals.

Alan's father was quite different from his unhappy wife. He enjoyed a modest financial success as the manager of a wholesale china firm. He was easy-going, comfortable with himself, and popular with young and old. His granddaughters, who met him only once, remember the twinkle in his eye as they responded to the warmth of his personality. On that occasion they met grandmother Brown and instinctively reacted against her cold indifference. The elder granddaughter, Barbara, peppering her phrases with expletives, summed her up as "an awful old bitch, I don't know why. I think she was born a bitch. I saw her only once or twice. But her sisters were pets and Grandfather was a darling — and a saint to put up with her!" In those days divorce was not lightly undertaken. In any case, George Brown was able to ride over the rough patches in his marriage. A less patient and more ambitious man might have given up.

Alan Brown's determination and cruelty, quite often deliberate, stemmed from his mother. From his father flowed the warmth and humanity that Alan displayed at home but which he rarely showed professionally except with his small patients. He was often amused by their remarks and when he was in a good mood he delighted in teasing them. Then shouts of laughter could be heard coming from the examining room.

His early childhood was marred by frequent colds and other minor complaints that he passed along to his younger siblings, much to his mother's annoyance. Recognizing the importance of good hygiene, she insisted that her children wash their hands with soap before their meals, constantly telling them that germs would not have a chance to slip down their throats with their food if their hands were clean. One day before supper, when Alan was three or four, she found him scrubbing his hands in a basin, the piece of soap almost rubbed into extinction. Disgusted, he turned towards her and complained, "This germ won't come out. I still have a sore throat."

He was a handsome child with fine, regular features, light brown hair and an engaging smile. As he was small for his age, he soon learned to be aggressive in order to defend himself against the bigger boys at

23

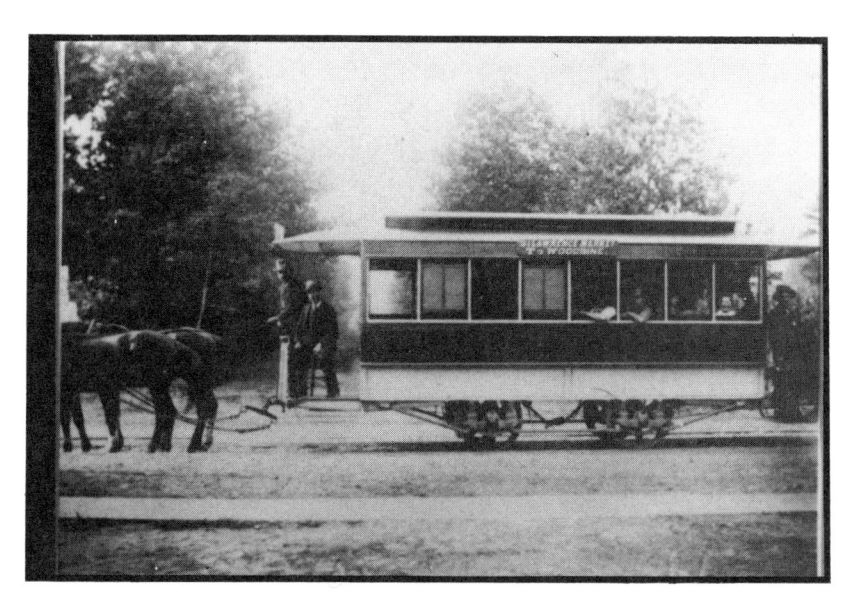

*Transportation when Alan was a boy: St. Lawrence Market to Woodbine
(Courtesy Toronto Archives)*

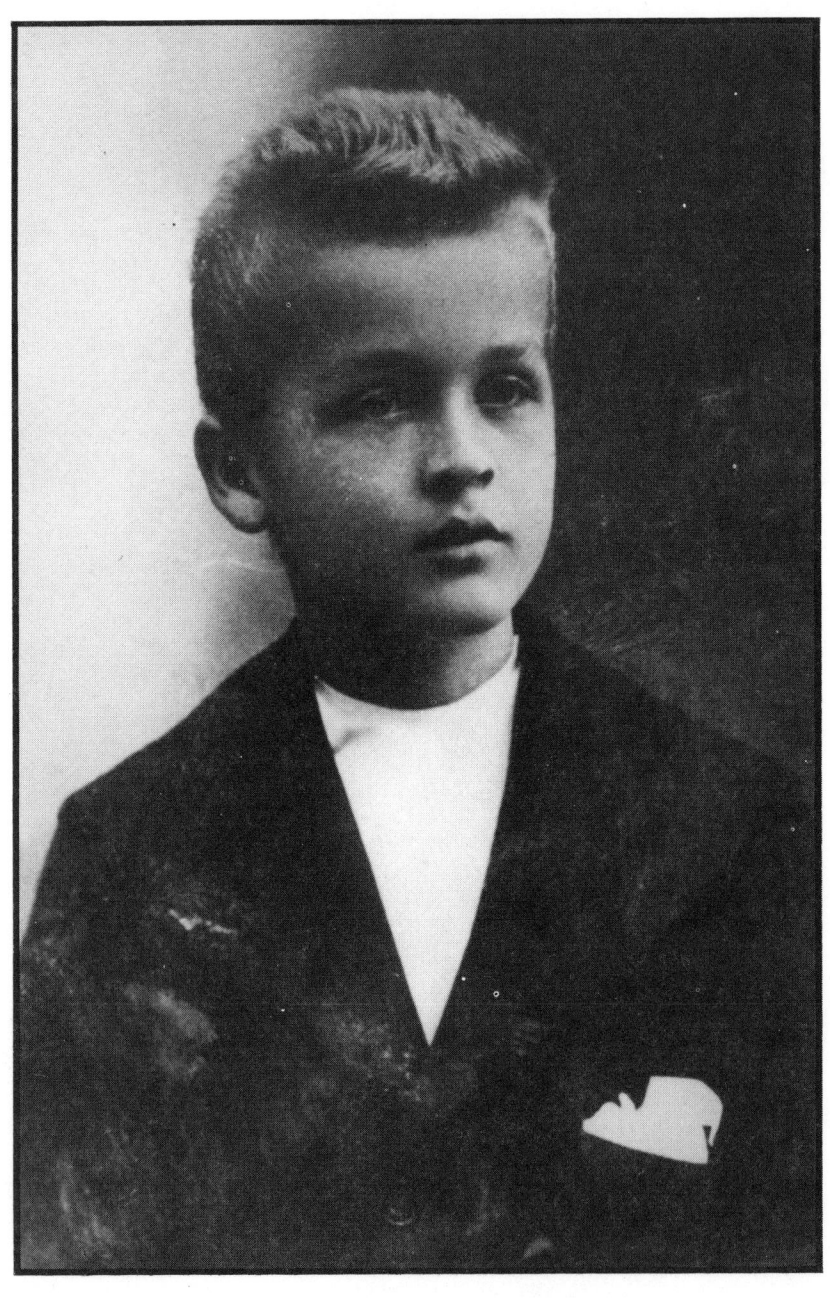

Alan Brown on Howland Avenue, Toronto, about 1897

his first school. This was a one-room building with twenty-four children in various grades who were taught by an adenoidal young man who had a perpetual cold; Alan wished he had had the courage to advise him on the virtues of hand washing. He was quick to learn and he loved to show off at home before his adoring younger brothers Clinton and Donald and his little sister Margery. They followed him around vying for his attention. Sometimes he would escape their pestering by hiding with a book and a snack among the leafy branches of the apple tree in their backyard, until their distant shouts enticed him back to join in their games.

In 1895 when Alan was eight years old the Browns moved to a rented semi-detached house at 155 Howland Avenue in Toronto. His mother, who dominated the family, sent her two oldest children, Alan and Clinton, to the Model School. She dressed them in the Little Lord Fauntleroy suits in vogue at the time due to the popularity of Frances Hodgson Burnett's books for children: knee-length velvet breeches with matching jacket and lace-trimmed collar with a big floppy silk bow. The other boys at the Model School in their ordinary cotton shirts, wool sweaters and sombre tweed breeches, gleefully swooped down on the two little boys in their finery. They were teased mercilessly and they begged their mother to let them wear ordinary clothes to school. After she had decided that plain clothes would cause less work for her, she finally relented.

During the late Victorian era and in the subsequent reign of Edward Vll, Toronto society was characterized by its respect for the monarchy, titles, old families and wealth — in that order. Most citizens of Canada had sailed from the British Isles bringing with them a reverence for "the mother country" and its traditions, some so pretentious as to be laughable today. Formal social visits were made on designated days often around eleven o'clock in the morning. With luck, the lady of the house would be out doing her own calls; the only function then required was the dropping of an embossed, engraved calling card on a silver tray on the hostess's hall table as proof that the convention had been observed. Some families weren't quite so silly. On the days they "received" they were usually at home to welcome their guests. These affectations, begun in the Victorian era, continued into the twentieth century and had become *de rigueur* by the time the Boer War ended in 1902 and the Klondike gold rush was in full swing. Meanwhile, the favoured few, steamer trunks packed with ball gowns and tail coats, sailed in style to Europe and "the old country" in the luxurious transatlantic passenger ships of the Cunard Line.

Everyone knew everybody of importance in the small Edwardian city that was Toronto. Climbing the social ladder was a serious game and snobbery was its name. Mr. and Mrs. Richard Hobbs played it with flair. One of their eleven children, Constance, was later to marry Alan Brown. In 1909 the Hobbs family was living at 4 Wellesley Place where the parents "received" in the afternoon on the second and fourth Monday of each month.

At Jarvis Collegiate in 1902, Alan played lacrosse, rugby, baseball and hockey. He was a good all-round athlete with one major handicap, according to a close school friend, Robert Mills[3] who was on the Jarvis football team when Alan was both its captain and its quarterback. Years later Mills laughed about it as he confided to his young cousin, Helen Reid, a student of Alan Brown, who reports:

> Bob said Alan was a hopeless quarterback; he was so timid he could never make up his mind what play to call next. Now Bob was very good at drawing cartoons. He told me that he had done a series of ten depicting "the little wimp" in action on the football field. Alan was not bossy or arrogant then. In fact he had seen and even thought these cartoons were funny at the time. But years later when they were grown men and Alan was concerned with his professional dignity, he demanded, "I want those cartoons and I'm going to get them." Bob replied, "Oh no, you're not! I'm keeping them." Quietly Alan enlisted friends to help him, suggesting they ask Bob to show the set of cartoons to them and then persuade him to let them "borrow" one or two. Little by little, over the course of several years, Alan managed to get almost all of them!

None, alas, has survived. However, the subject of one of the cartoons is well known; his daughter Barbara Alan Brown Kelley describes it:

> One day at U of T when he was practising with his team, one of the big players picked him up under his arm and ran him down the field for a touchdown. Father laughed as he told me the story but said he was furious at the time.

Shortly after this "touchdown" he broke a finger. The clumsiness of his cast made him realize how important sensitive hands were to a

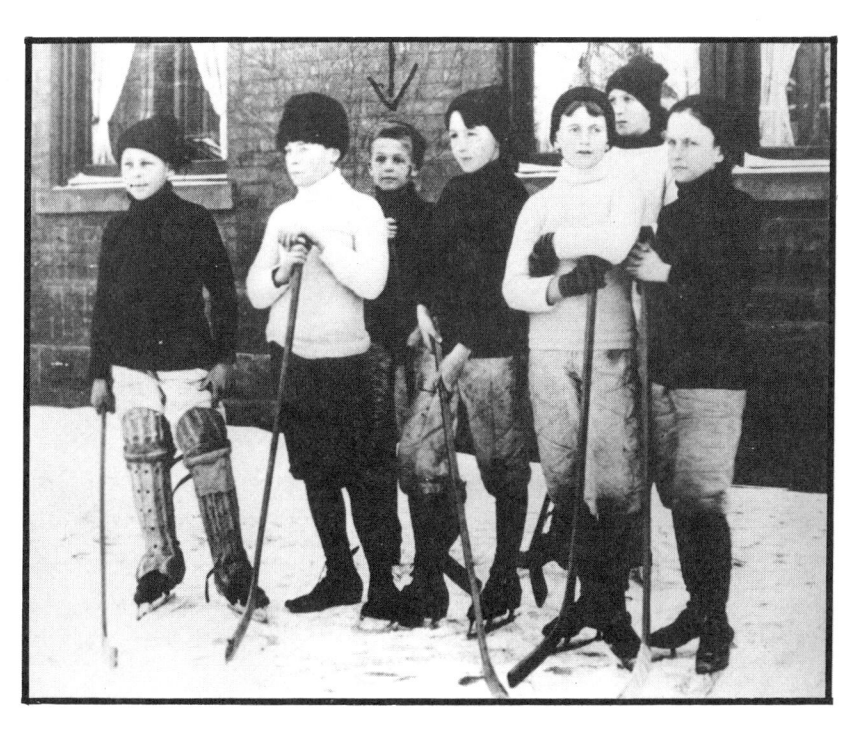

Alan and his hockey team, about 1900: Flett, Kingston, Brown, Rost, Band, Follet, Dalton (HSC Archives)

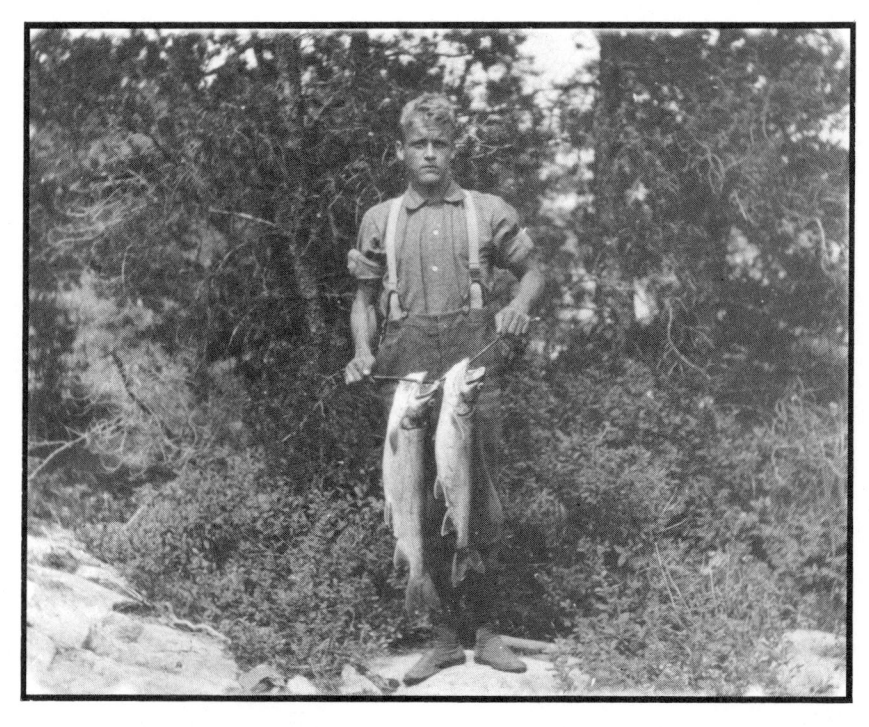

Alan displays his catch, about 1904

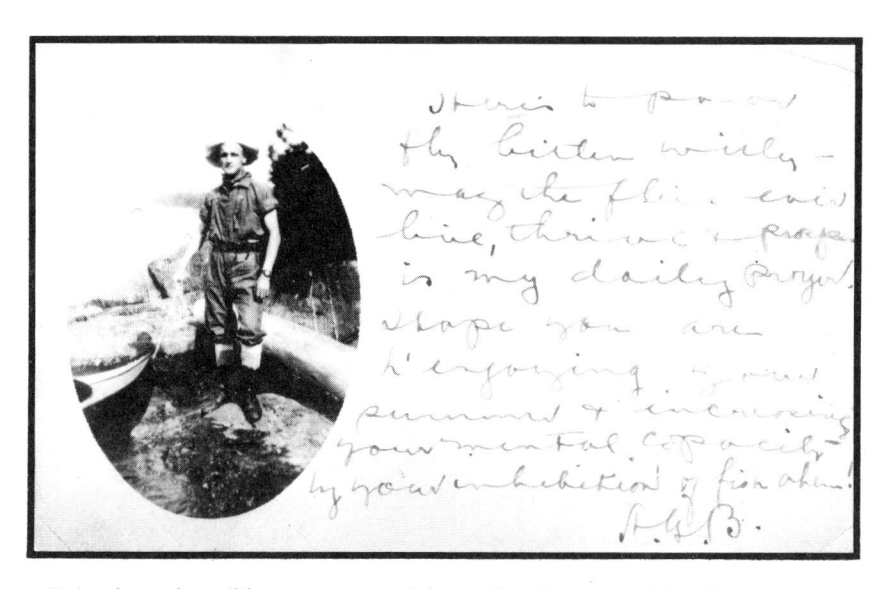

Voice from the wilderness: postcard from Alan Brown to Miss Constance Hobbs in 1908

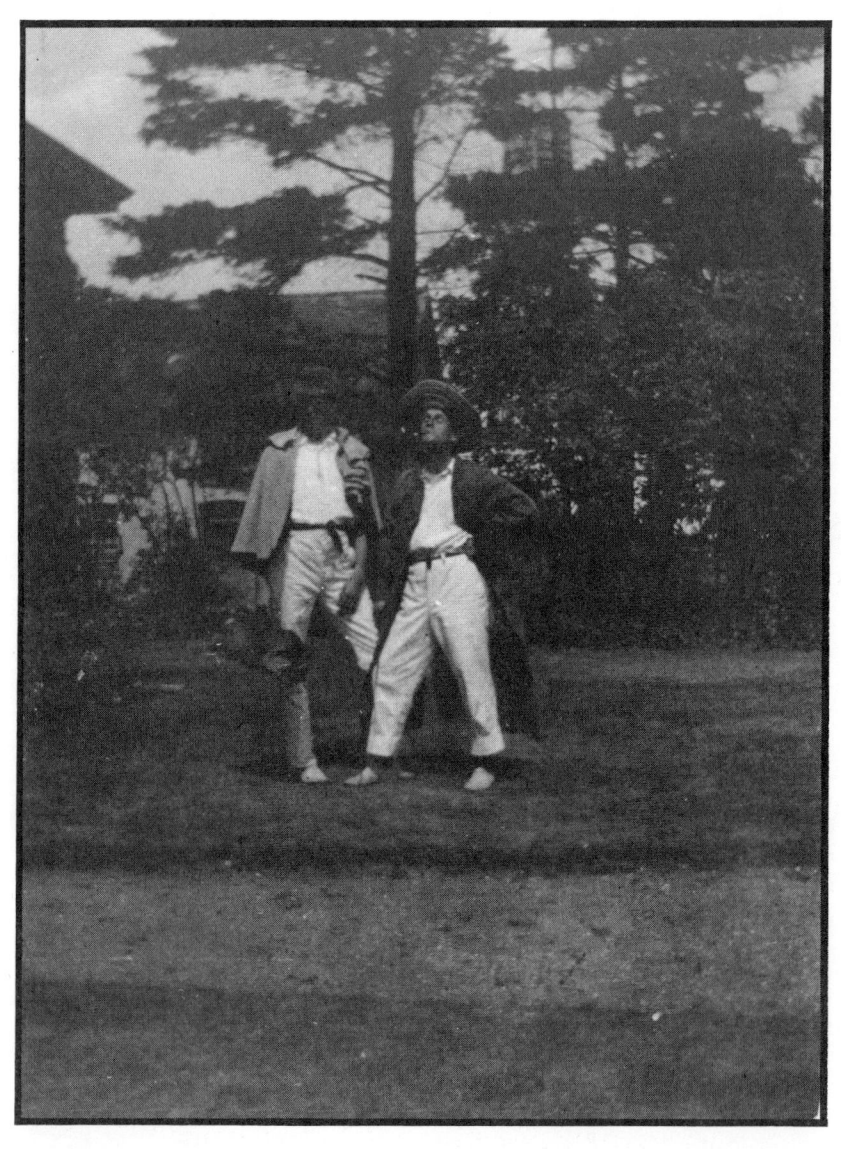

Alan clowning with pipe and Charlie Dalton at the Hobbs farm, London, Ontario, 1909

Casual courting: Charles Dalton, Beatrice Hobbs, Alan Brown and Constance Hobbs at the Hobbs farm, London, Ontario, 1909

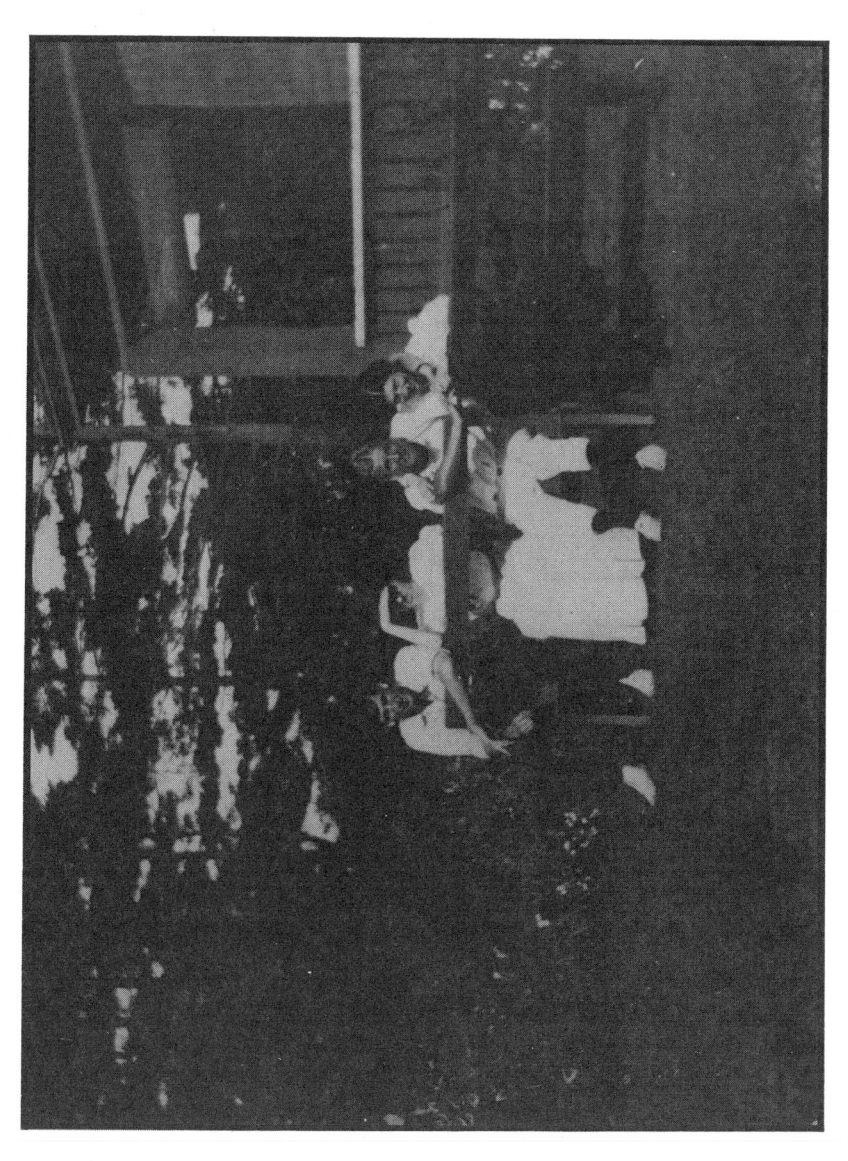

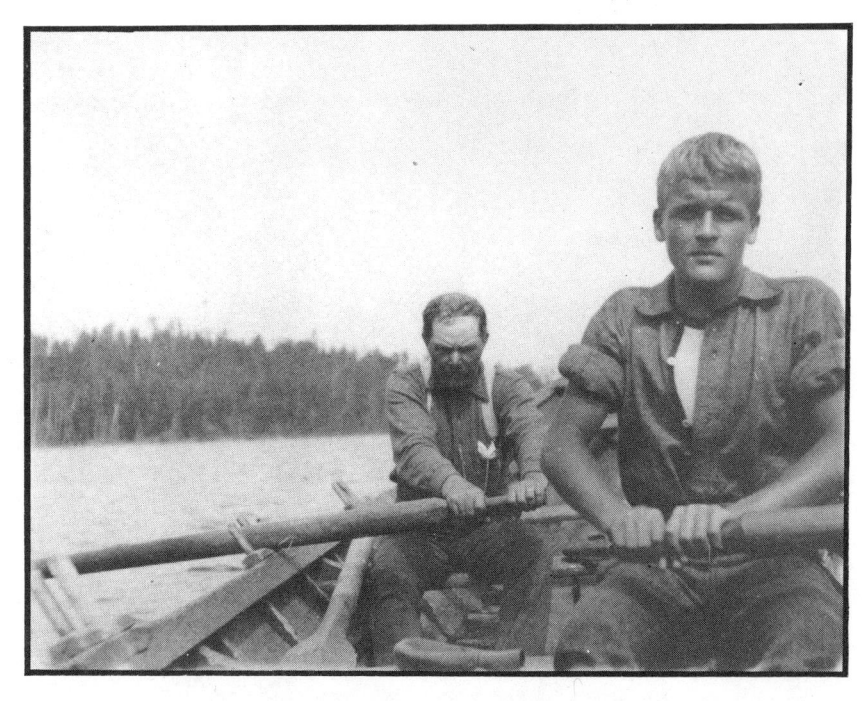

Alan manning the oars with a friend

doctor. He decided he would have to give up the game. He became manager of the team instead, and was later elected to the University of Toronto Athletic Association. In addition, he was a member of the Alpha Delta fraternity. After he graduated in 1909 he was elected to Alpha Omicron, an honorary fraternity and a reading club that often met at the Browns'.

He spent his first university summer holiday on a farm near London, Ontario, where he pitched manure and hay. His niece, Elizabeth Fisher Lawson, recalls Alan's lamenting the pain when opening his hands after the first day of hard labour in the fields. Once the blisters had hardened into callouses he began to enjoy the outdoor work.

Constance Hobbs spent part of the summer on the family farm where Alan was working. Her father, Richard Hobbs, had a hardware store in London and his own manufacturing company, Consolidated Plate Glass, on Bathurst Street in Toronto. During the two months Alan worked on the farm he gradually fell in love with Connie. For her it happened the moment she laid eyes on him. She was an uninhibited and attractive chatterbox who amused him with her outrageous remarks and her ability to mimic. Respect for prominent figures in Toronto's social and political set was tossed aside as she parodied them, or gleefully imitated the oddities of the family's friends and relatives. Her barbs spared no one when she had the urge to let them fly. "She couldn't stand Raymond Massey who lived next door to them on Wellesley Place," Nancy Alan Brown Mayer recalls, "and she and some of my aunts used to climb the fence and spit at him. She was very witty and could imitate absolutely anybody." Her audacity increased with the years. When she mimicked the long orations of their marble-mouthed, sanctimonious minister at Deer Park United, Alan laughed till he cried "uncle". Connie was barely sixteen that summer when they met on the farm. He was fascinated by her. She made him laugh with her small talk, a social skill he never mastered. Instead, he covered up his deficiency by drawing on his collection of jokes. Connie had a closer relationship with her father than with her mother. "Grandfather Hobbs adored children; grandmother didn't. But domestic help was plentiful for those who could afford it, so grandmother had lots of babies." Another granddaughter said, "She wasn't the slightest bit maternal. As soon as decency allowed, she passed her babies over to a nanny." After marriage to Richard, Anne Osborne Hobbs persuaded her half sister, Sarah, to be their housekeeper. The Hobbs children were devoted to their Aunt Sarah. Her interest and affection compensated for their mother's serene indifference. Mrs. Hobbs remained aloof throughout her life, treating her children as politely as any of her casual acquaintances.

Chapter 3
Internship, Post-graduate Training and Marriage

AFTER HIS graduation with honours in 1909 from the University of Toronto Medical School and winning the Silver Medal his mother scorned, Alan Brown was admitted to a one-year internship at The Hospital for Sick Children. Over the years since its opening in 1875 — one year earlier than Johns Hopkins — the HSC had achieved a fine reputation in North America. Alan Brown was to add to its lustre. Interning with him in the old College Street building, Gordon Gallie became an obstetrician attached to the Toronto General Hospital on University Avenue. Many years later, their close and lasting friendship was instrumental in the saving of Brown's life.

In Edwardian times and throughout the 1920s the dress of the HSC interns was formal and highly impractical for work in the wards: starched, white cotton suits with brass buttons that demanded a daily polish, and high, stiff collars fastened with collar studs, and bow ties. More uncomfortable and unsuitable clothing cannot be imagined. Thus attired, interns worked long hot hours beside their nursing colleagues similarily clad.

Once children became ill there was little medication available other than aspirin and morphine. Vaccines, sulphonamides, penicillin and other antibiotics were not to appear for another twenty to thirty years. Intravenous therapy for dehydration and cardiovascular shock was still in its infancy although it had been tried experimentally in England as early as the end of the nineteenth century. It was not commonly used

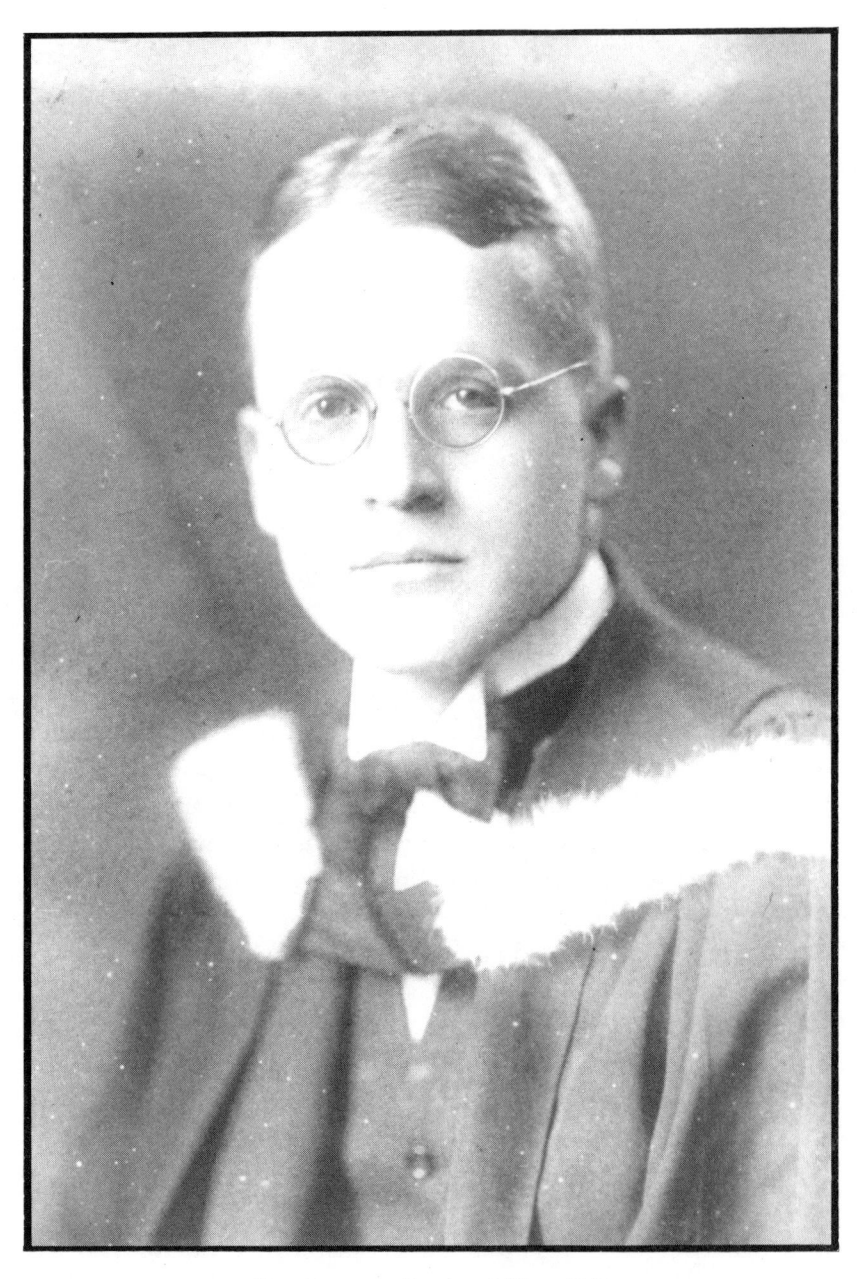

Alan Brown, silver medallist, 1909

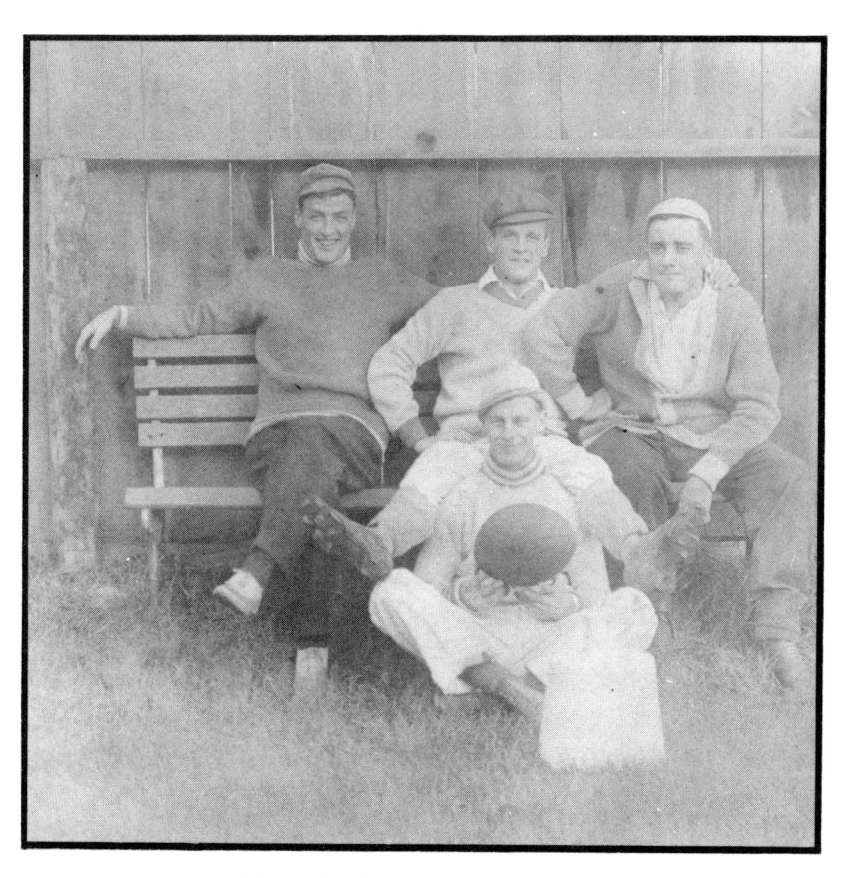

Hospital for Sick Children (HSC) interns at play, 1909: Gordon Gallie, Alan Brown, Ross Jamieson and Ted Morgan

in the HSC wards before the advent of Alan Brown. Childhood infectious diseases were rampant and poor hygiene spread cross-infection throughout the wards. Measles, scarlet fever, mumps or chicken pox could race through the wards from a single patient whose infection became apparent only after admission. "We used to go round the wards and inject the children with 20cc of horse serum to protect them against scarlet fever."[1] Any infant who sickened with whooping cough rarely recovered. A child hospitalized with diphtheria, pneumonia or meningitis had less than a fifty percent chance of survival. "The number of children who used to die of these diseases is just incomprehensible now. People today haven't the slightest idea of the tremendous amount of disability and death that occurred from infections in the days before we had, first, immunization and then antibiotics."[2] Parents brought their children to hospital only as a last resort. They were terrified by rumours of the great number of deaths in the wards and so they delayed bringing in their children for treatment. When they did it was often too late.

Alan Brown was angry that so many children were dying. As an HSC intern he was shocked by the lack of cleanliness in the wards; he knew from his upbringing that the first step to good hygiene was frequent handwashing. Gastroenteritis and the consequent dehydration was the biggest contributor to the high mortality rates. Malnutrition was common, causing rotting teeth or rickets from vitamin D deficiency. Unpasteurized milk was responsible for the prevalence of bovine tuberculosis and other bacterial disorders. But in some areas progress had been made. For example, as early as the 1880s the HSC's surgeons had been recognized throughout North America for straightening bone malformations, particularly of the legs (club foot, hip dislocations and nutritional deformities such as bowlegs and knock-knees).

During his one-year internship at HSC, Alan and Connie continued to see one other but the grinding hours an intern was obliged to work did not allow much free time. They had little money to spend on amusements but enjoyed wandering around the parks and the beaches of the city. During the summer months Alan spent two weeks as intern at the HSC's Lakeside Home for Little Children on Centre Island at Lighthouse Point. Here children convalesced after their discharge from their time at HSC. When not on duty he slept in the staff quarters — a long row of small, one-storey wooden buildings that today might, euphemistically, rate as town houses. These were joined by raised wooden sidewalks above the scrub and sand. The surrounding area was the joy of the staff's children for it held, to their delight, hundreds of midget toads for their entertainment.

Once or twice during Alan's stint at the Lakeside Home, Connie rode over on the ferry and Alan took her canoeing through the lagoons of Toronto's islands. She didn't much like boats and water but adored the man who did. She could swim, but not well. The long skirts of that day were not exactly an asset as she tried to clamber in or out without upsetting the canoe. Once seated, however, the romance of being paddled through the winding waters overcame her aversion; but she was always relieved when they returned to dry land when Alan would spring from the canoe, brush off his knees and bend down to offer her a helping hand.

On one occasion, her adoration for Alan was tested. She had reluctantly accompanied him to the hospital, just for a minute to check the results of an autopsy, as he said. Connie hated hospitals but she took him at his word and sat down to wait. He became so engrossed with his thoughts that he forgot about her and left the hospital by another door. Half way home he realized his blunder and hastily retraced his steps — too late to scotch her fury.

When his internship ended in the spring of 1910 he immediately began a three-year residency in New York City at the Babies' Hospital, then on the corner of 55th and Lexington. There he studied under two small men, who were nevertheless the paediatric giants of their time in North America : Dr. Emmett Holt and Dr. Abraham Jacobi, the father of American paediatrics. At that time Dr. Holt was in his early fifties, a little man with short white hair, always immaculate and as formal in speech as he was in dress. No one ever joked with him and his relationship with his staff was pleasant but formal. His unbiased attitude toward women was unusual in the days when they were still denied the right to vote. Until 1912 most of the residents he chose were women; he thought they would make better paediatricians than men. The Superintendent of the Babies' Hospital, who was also the director of the nursing and intern staff, was a Toronto graduate, Miss Mary Agnes Smith, whose advice Holt sought before filling any residency post. Due to her influence, every chief male resident of the Babies' Hospital from 1912 to 1920 was a Canadian.[3]

An impatient but courteous dictator, it never once crossed Holt's mind that anyone might disobey an order, and no one ever did. He was an excellent clinician and teacher and Alan was impressed with both his knowledge and his methods. Following Holt, as he made rounds with his staff, Brown learned a pattern that he was to use throughout his thirty-six years at HSC. Holt's abrupt comments, questions and brilliant diagnoses, as he moved from bed to bed, were to have a lasting influence on Brown and on the way he later conducted his own hospital rounds.

Intellectual excitement as much as hard work filled the young doctor's days and nights. The stimulation of living in cosmopolitan New York with its gaudy bustle was a revelation to Alan Brown. He became acquainted with Nathan Strauss, the great philanthropist and owner of Macy's Department Store, a handsome old man, always elegantly dressed, his white hair and beard neatly groomed. He was both cultured and compassionate, with an urgent sense of his duty towards the less fortunate. Brown was awed by the way Strauss and the wealthy Jewish community quite naturally assumed responsibility for newly arrived immigrants of the same religion and race. Strauss also showed his great concern for children. He initiated and personally subsidized The New York City Milk Fund, a service to provide milk for children in the slum schools. He befriended the young doctor and included him at several social functions attended by the Guggenheim brothers and other representatives of New York society and philanthropy. He also introduced Alan to opera, but the occasion seems to have made little impression on him for there is no evidence he ever attended an opera again.

One night in New York when he was on call in Emergency, an adult psychiatric patient was delivered to the Babies' Hospital by mistake. Alan's daughter described the incident: "Father was the intern ordered to go with this nut to the appropriate hospital. Now, Dad was quite small and the two of them were locked up in the back of the ambulance. The man was handcuffed but he was still big and powerful. He was easily able to overpower Dad as they struggled together in the swaying ambulance." Many years later Alan Brown said to Barbara, "Thank God we arrived when we did! He had me down on the floor with his hands around my throat. I couldn't breathe and I thought, 'I'm gone, this is it, I'm gone'. Then suddenly the sirens ceased and the ambulance jerked to a stop. The doors opened and cool air rushed in with the attendants who 'wrenched the patient's hands away just in the nick of time. There was nothing I could have done. He was bigger and stronger — and paranoid.' "

Shortly before he finished his trainIng at the Babies' Hospital he survived another encounter with death. No doubt about it, New York City was dangerous even then. Boarding at the house of an elderly couple, he was working late one summer night on a paper he was writing with Dr. Holt on the treatment for infants with hereditary syphilis. The door bell rang. It was two o'clock in the morning. The night was stifling and Brown was working at his desk in the nude. He didn't want the owners wakened and hastily grabbed his dressing gown just as the bell sounded again. He flew downstairs from the attic, his robe floating open behind him. It snagged as he rounded the last newel post and was ripped off just as he opened the door. Confronting him was a huge black man who lunged at the naked man and flung him to the floor. In shock at first, his vocal cords registered only a squawk then, at last, a loud shout seconds before the intruder knocked him out cold. The landlord and his wife heard the cry. She rang the police while her husband held his automatic on the suddenly submissive attacker until the police burst in the door minutes later. Embarrassment over his nakedness worried Alan Brown more than his throbbing head. But he laughed about it when he told his daughter many years later, "The man was simply huge and I didn't have a stitch on."

Early in September 1913, Brown returned to Toronto briefly before booking his passage for Europe on the Cunard Line to study under Professors Heinrich Finkelstein, L.F. Meyer and Adalbert Czerny. Just as he was exposed to the best of Jewish philanthropy in Nathan Strauss and his associates in New York City, he was to be favourably impressed by the best of Jewish medicine in Berlin and Munich. Because of these close Jewish associations Alan Brown was unusual among Toronto's middle class. He was not anti-Semitic, unlike many of his friends, relatives and colleagues at that time.

In the Children's Hospital of Berlin University Czerny and Finkelstein taught courses in biochemistry and nutrition that were famous throughout Europe. Dr. Finkelstein, also Director of The Infant Asylum and City Orphanage in Berlin, was an expert clinician and a creative nutritionist. He and Dr. Meyer developed Eiweissmilch, the high protein milk made with egg white, a variation of which Brown was later to produce and prescribe for his patients whose condition did not improve with lactic acid milk.

The autocratic methods of instruction that Alan Brown observed in class and clinic both in North America and Europe, convinced him that the only way to introduce and maintain new procedures and treatments was to travel along the same road. Following the example of those from whom he had learned, with dedicated ruthlessness he pushed the HSC into its medical future and added to its renown throughout the medical world.

Some German medical practices he could not accept. He was appalled that many German surgeons performed tonsillectomies without giving their little patients any anaesthetic. This horrified and infuriated him. In the Germany before World War I there were other disturbing sights. One day when he was walking with one of his professors in Berlin, Brown asked, "What is that terrible stench?" Bitterly the professor replied, "Feldgasses."[4] Flouting the Geneva Convention of the League of Nations, the Germans were developing and testing mustard and other gases to be used against an enemy in the event of war.

So impressed had Alan Brown been with Dr. Finkelstein, the man and the teacher, that he corresponded with him regularly between the two world wars. When Dr. Finkelstein and his wife fled from Hitler's Germany to Chile in 1933, the year Adolph Hitler came to power, Brown sent them money and kept their correspondence alive. When Finkelstein died in 1942 Brown continued assisting his widow with additional funds and offers of help at any time in the future should she need it.

In December 1913, Alan Brown sailed home on leave to enjoy Christmas with Connie and her family before their marriage on the seventeenth of January 1914. Alan was gradually enveloped by the Hobbs family while he slowly became estranged from his own. The silver medal episode of 1909 had severely strained his relationship with his mother. He rarely visited his parents although they lived in the same district. They were not invited to the wedding. His sister Margery was invited but had to decline. She had already married and was living in the southern States, too far away to justify the expense of the journey. As for Clinton, he and Alan had little in common; whether he was present at the wedding is not known. Donald had always admired and looked up to his older brother and would certainly have attended. Alan's best man was Ted Morgan and his ushers included Bruce Robertson, George Strathy, Ruggles George and Whiteford Bell. Among Connie's attendants were Helen Warren, Eva Haney, Marjorie Rathbun and her youngest sister, Yvonne Hobbs, as maid of honour.

The honeymoon introduced Connie to voyaging by luxury liner, and she was hooked for life. She was to criss-cross the ocean many times in the years ahead. On this first occasion the Browns booked tourist class but they cast the ship's rules to the winds when a wealthy friend in first class invited them up to her luxurious quarters for tea. Such an opportunity was not to be missed. There were strict rules to prevent the passengers from one class mixing with those in another but, as he later told his daughter, "We went up anyway and your mother thought she was sailing to Europe in high style." Alan Brown began to laugh at another memory. "After my previous six months in Berlin, I was confident my German was pretty good so when we arrived in the Munich train station I spoke to the porter in German. I asked him to take us 'wenden' to a taxi. He looked a bit puzzled but politely said, 'Sir, I think I understand you better if you speak in English.' What I'd really said was, 'Please turn us over in a taxi.' "[5]

Keeping their small rented rooms tidy left Connie time to explore each city they visited while Alan was studying stools in the Bender and Hobein Laboratories, working and observing in hospital clinics in Berlin, Munich and Vienna. Connie adored antiques of any kind — jewellery, furniture, china — and went window shopping almost every day. There was one shop in her Munich neighbourhood where she often stopped for a chat with the owner. He spoke very little English and Connie not much German other than "bitte schön, danke zehr, gemütlich, schrechlich." By miming with face and hands they amused each other and persuaded themselves they understood one another most of the time. She bought a couple of small, delicately wrought mosaic brooches. Fifty years later her granddaughter Ann, on a visit to Munich, entered the same shop and discovered pins similar to those her grandmother had bought so many years before. She bought two, one for herself and one for her grandmother who was delighted to learn the shop had survived both world wars and was still selling the same exquisite jewellery. The son of the proprietor whom Connie had known was the current owner. He said his father had died several years before Ann's visit.

As Connie looked at her granddaughter's gift, memories of those five months flooded through her mind. She began to describe to Ann the highlights of their life in Germany. She had little respect for the facts if they failed to match her imagination. Ann was enchanted. While her grandfather's energy and intellect concentrated on medicine and the hospital, her grandmother, as she talked, lived in the memory of those days with Alan in Germany just before the Great War.

As Connie strolled through the streets of the city she saw many photographs of Kaiser Wilhelm, King of Prussia and Emperor of the Germanies, in his full military regalia. He was a handsome man with a carefully trimmed beard. Connie thought he looked like his cousin George V. She loved to watch the many parades and to hear the military bands with their blaring brass and crashing cymbals. Although she was caught up in the emotions of the crowds she had misgivings as she watched the German soldiers goose-stepping along the avenues in their high polished boots, shouldering heavy rifles and led by sword-swinging officers. Once she saw the Kaiser reviewing the troops. He was resplendent in dress uniform, the medals across his chest gleaming in the sun. She cynically wondered what acts of bravery he had committed to win them. Then came her memories of wasted lives, devastation and the degradation suffered by both armies in the trenches during those four years. Ann forgotten, Connie sat quietly, lost in her thoughts.

Suddenly, shaking her head, she looked up and began to clown again. She mimicked the shopkeepers and ordinary people she had known then, and laughed out loud at her audacious portrayals of the stuffy and pompous medical men and their meek little wives whom she and Alan encountered at the boring social occasions they were obliged to attend. Connie was a natural storyteller and actress. Ann was a captive audience. She listened and watched as her grandmother by gesture and speech paraded before her the people and the places she had known long ago. Ann felt the excitement, frustrations and forebodings that her grandmother experienced in Germany during the uneasy months before the Great War exploded in August of 1914. During those days her grandfather, steeped in the urgency of learning, was oblivious to the unmistakable evidence around him of impending war.

Chapter 4

World War I and Alan Brown's Battles

With some relief, Alan and Connie Brown sailed home from Germany in the spring of 1914 as the Kaiser was rattling his sabre. In June, the Archduke Ferdinand, Emperor Franz Joseph's heir to the Austro-Hungarian Empire, was assassinated in Sarajevo and the fuse was ignited: "the war to end all wars" was about to erupt. Few saw it coming. During that uneasy summer ordinary men and women led their usual lives unaware of the gathering storm that would lay waste the life they knew, in some cases forever.

Hostilities began in the Balkan states and spread quickly across Europe. The Allied forces included Great Britain, France, Belgium, Russia and Japan. The opposing Central Powers included Germany and the Austro-Hungarian and Ottoman Empires. By early September, World War I was well under way. Over the next four years the Allied armies lost more than five million men, the enemy a comparable number. Ten million men — twice the population of Canada at the time.

During one encounter alone — the first Battle of the Somme in 1916 — more than seventy-four thousand lives were lost. The brunt of the front-line leadership on the Western Front fell on the young subalterns. Easily identified from the other ranks by their distinctive uniforms, the carnage among junior officers was disproportionately high as they led their troops across "no man's land" to attack the enemy trenches. With the death of these well-educated, ambitious, peacetime leaders, the world lost a precious generation.

The City in Wartime
By the end of 1914 there were few who continued to believe the war would be over in six months. Hospitals became short-staffed as nurses and doctors enlisted. Toronto began to shed its parochialism. Its citizens lost their narrow focus and saw the rest of the world through a wide-angled lens. The Boer War had scarcely disturbed their complacency in spite of the enthusiasm with which they had entered into it. A World War awakened them. Newspapers posted daily casualty lists in their windows as the public closely followed the progress of the battles their men were fighting. When the Germans, flouting the Geneva Convention, used mustard gas, public resolve hardened.

In Canada skilled workers of both sexes toiled in munitions factories, sometimes round the clock. To pay for the war the Federal Government introduced Income Tax for the first time in the nation's history, as a "temporary measure". The unskilled worked for the Red Cross as drivers or bandage rollers, knitted balaclavas or socks and packed food parcels. Many other volunteer groups sprang up to contribute. One young woman,[1] trained as a volunteer nurse's aid, was sent to the military convalescent hospital in Whitby. She went off to her war with two horses in tow. "Nobody thought it unusual and the hospital was happy about it. There were lots of convalescing officers to help me exercise them."

The glamour of danger was seductive, the consequences unforeseen. An air force pilot, from the training base just outside Toronto, was madly in love with a young woman who lived on Glengowan Road. Impatient with the slow delivery of the Royal Mail he used to bring her his letters himself — in his air force one-seater. He tied a tiny parachute to each of his letters and dipped his wings as he dropped them over her house. The neighbourhood children were agog at the sight of the toy missiles as they drifted down from the 'plane. One day he did not return to base: he had misjudged the height of some hydro wires.

Paediatric Pioneer
In 1914 Alan Brown was twenty-seven years old. He had four years of postgraduate paediatric training behind him. Returning to Canada during that smouldering summer before war began, he was impatient to

embark upon his life's work: to dedicate all his energy, experience and skill to saving the lives of infants and children and to promoting their good health. No other physician practising in Canada at that time had studied the diseases and the special needs of children as intensely and thoroughly as he had. He was returning to his country to become Canada's first academically and clinically qualified paediatrician.

Early "Paediatricians"

Before Alan Brown's return from his postgraduate training, the practice of paediatrics in Canada had been carried on in a haphazard fashion. Those interested in treating children did so whenever they could spare the time from their adult practice, their main source of income. There were so-called departments of paediatrics in several Canadian cities before 1920, but those who headed them had had no formal paediatric training, except for Alan Brown. In 1895 Dr. René Fortier was appointed Professor of Paediatrics at Laval University in Quebec City; Dr. I.W. Wood at Queen's University in 1905; Dr. A.D. Blackader at McGill in 1912; Dr. W.J. Tilman at University of Western Ont. in 1913; and Dr. Alan Brown, the Hospital for Sick Children's Physician-in-Chief and Associate Professor of Medicine at the University of Toronto in 1919. The earliest children's hospitals were the Hospital for Sick Children, Toronto, 1875; the Childrens' Memorial Hospital, Montreal, 1902; L'Hôpital Ste. Justine pour les Enfants, Montreal, 1907; the Children's Hospital, Winnipeg, 1909; the Children's Hospital, Halifax, 1910.[2]

With the exception of Alan Brown, the early professors of paediatrics were all self-taught, with no formal training in the diseases and special needs of children. Dr. Blackader, for example, as a medical student had majored in pharmacology and therapeutics, but because of his interest in children he lectured in paediatrics at McGill and was one of the founders of the American Pediatric Society in 1888. He was the first in Canada to work for the recognition of paediatrics as a specialty in its own right. Self-taught paediatricians soon became anomalies in the medical profession as Alan Brown's and, later, Alton Goldbloom's students began to spread across the country as professors of paediatrics at other Canadian universities. Dr. Goldbloom had followed Brown's postgraduate road to The Babies' Hospital in New York where he too studied under Emmett Holt. He returned to Montreal to open a private practice in 1920.

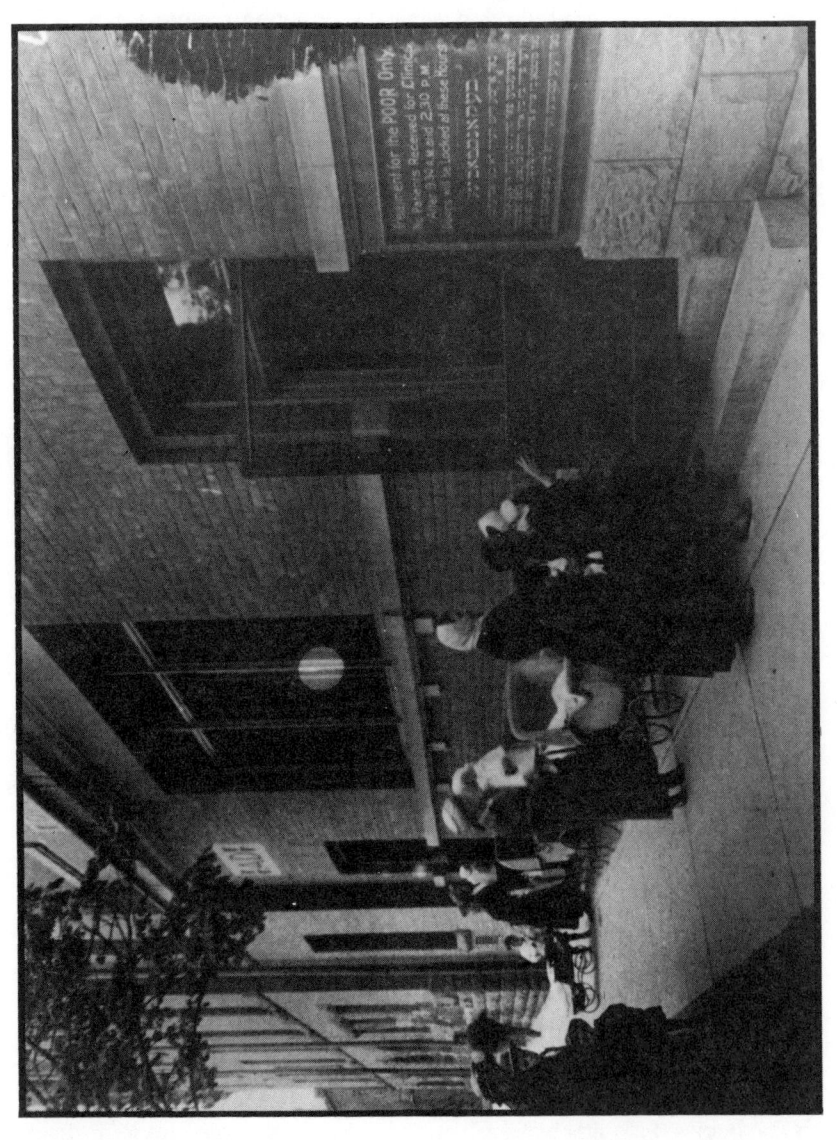

1915, Alan Brown on HSC staff: sign at entrance to Out Patients reads: "Treatment for the Poor only". Hebrew version follows. (Courtesy Dr. Frederick Weinberg)

The Dawn of Specialty Medicine

The training of specialists was resisted by general practitioners who guarded their right to treat every medical and surgical problem presented to them. Medical practice was a dog fight — everyone fighting for and jealous of his own turf. Doctors interested in specializing learned by trial and error. Nobody was formally trained in paediatrics and GPs sometimes knew no more than grandmothers about the treatment of sick children. When Alan Brown returned to Toronto there was no formal training in surgery even for those who had decided to concentrate on it. At several major Canadian hospitals, departments of surgery were staffed entirely by general practitioners. Their "surgical" experience had been limited to the dissection of cadavers when they were medical students in the anatomy department. In large hospitals they often received initial surgical guidance by assisting experienced general practice surgeons at operations, but in the small towns, where many set up in practice without any earlier surgical experience, they were on their own from the beginning. If they had the courage to remove a gall bladder or an appendix, they simply did so. More than twenty years were to elapse before Alan Brown's colleague, Edward Gallie, followed his example by organizing the country's first formal course for postgraduate students who wanted to specialize in surgery. Both Brown and Gallie had to overcome the opposition of the general practitioner who correctly foresaw a sizeable part of his practice usurped by the new specialist.

Hospital Doctors: Conscripted Volunteers

Before World War II, physicians and surgeons on hospital staffs were unpaid by the hospital and depended on their private practices to carry their professional and personal expenses. Interns were the exception. They at least received a stipend — enough to buy food or shelter but not both. For the privilege of being attached to a hospital, regular staff members were expected to spend many hours a week treating public patients wihout fee in the hospital clinics and wards. Before the advent of universal medical insurance this method of treating the hospital's patients was clearly necessary. At The Hospital for Sick Children there were no salaried physicians until 1946, when Brown recommended that Drs. Harry Ebbs and Nelles Silverthorne be hired full-time by the hospital. During the thirty-two years he served as Physician-in-Chief, Dr. Alan Brown received only $800 a year to use at his discretion for any unbudgeted expenses of the HSC Department of Medicine.[3] The situation at other teaching hospitals was similar. Those who taught in the Faculty of Medicine were not paid. The prestige they acquired from teaching positions attracted more than enough patients to their private practices to support all their professional and personal expenses.

Brown vs Baines

By 1915, after one year in private practice, Alan Brown considered his personal income adequate to make him financially self-sufficient. He was impatient to reach out to the hospital's public patients. With a characteristic sense of urgency bordering on aggression he expected to be warmly welcomed at The Hospital for Sick Children. After all, he had earlier served one year there as an intern and he was now returning as a full-fledged specialist paediatrician.

Fortified by the confidence his years of post-graduate training and paediatric experience had given him, Alan Brown was convinced he could lower the high mortality rate in the infant wards. In the early years of the twentieth century, until 1913, the infant mortality rate was so high that The Hospital for Sick Children did not admit patients under two years of age. Alan Brown's arrival was timely. The challenge he faced was formidable. "During the summers the infants used to die like flies — so many deaths at night that the interns wouldn't get up to pronounce them dead and so we lined them up in the linen closet — five or six little bodies every morning. It was terrible," Helen McCallum, RN, relates.

Confident of his reception, Alan Brown asked for an interview with Dr. Allen Baines, chief physician and a staff member since 1891. Baines made it quite clear that he did not need any more doctors. He did not want "any of these new-fangled paediatricians fooling around" in his hospital and he refused to appoint "this young whippersnapper,"[4] as he later described him to one of his residents, Ted Morgan. (Morgan had a close but sometimes uneasy relationship with Alan until it broke down completely after a shocking incident some thirty years later.)

Brown was angered but not discouraged by Baines' refusal to appoint him. He discussed his next move with his friend, Bruce Robertson, already on staff. He was the nephew of John Ross Robertson, a generous benefactor of the hospital for more than thirty years and Chairman of its Board of Trustees. Dr. Robertson spoke to his uncle of Brown's conviction that he could cut the mortality rate in the infants' wards by fifty percent within a year. "And I believe him," he said. Impressed by this statement, Robertson, in his capacity as Chairman of the Board, appointed Alan Brown to the HSC staff on a trial basis and assigned him one of the infants' wards where he was expected to fulfill his promise.

In many ways John Ross Robertson was very much like Alan Brown. He was not in the habit of consulting others about his decisions and he did not inform Allen Baines of Brown's provisional appointment. A day or two later Baines came on the ward one morning and found Brown making rounds. "What the hell are you doing here?" Brown turned to him and coolly said, "Baines, from now I'm running this ward and I'll thank you to respect my position."[5]

Alan Brown on Trial

On that first day in 1915, confident, determined and bursting with energy, he descended on "his" infants' ward. The attending nurses and doctors were stunned into immediate obedience by the whirlwind that swept through it. He demanded clean hands and sterilization of food, utensils and instruments. He brooked no dissension. There was no other way to prevent cross-infection. In an era when doctors practised "crisis" medicine, their time taken up by those who were already ill, Alan Brown practised preventive medicine on his small patients by strict hygienic measures, special diets designed for specific conditions, and ruthless removal of diseased body tissues — usually tonsils, teeth and appendix. Today people haven't the faintest idea of the amount of disability and death from infections before immunization and antibiotics. Alan Brown had a tremendous fight to establish his standards of cleanliness, medical care and diet. He had to be very tough. He didn't care what anybody thought. His decisions were final and he expected to be obeyed without question. His sense of urgency increased due to the war, then in full swing, as HSC staff departed to join the armed forces. In most cases he could not fill the gaps and had to demand more from those who remained.

War at the Front — and at Home

Alan Brown's close friend Bruce Robertson was one of the first to enlist. Torn by the sense of conflicting responsibilities, Alan asked Bruce for advice in deciding what he should do. Bruce was adamant. "As a surgeon I can save the lives of the wounded. Your wounded are here —

save the lives of the babies. This is where you are needed. Besides, a paediatrician is not exactly an asset in the trenches."[6]

Convinced by his friend's blunt argument, Alan Brown stayed with his infants. During those four years he fought his own battles on two fronts: against disease and the hostility of some of his staff. Although he treated and saved hundreds of children while their fathers served overseas, he had to face the resentment felt by some of the veterans returning to the HSC staff or attending his classes and clinics.

Alan Brown's Promise Fulfilled

Before the end of 1915, his first year on staff, he had stood the ward on its ear and had almost made good his boast. He had reduced the number of infant deaths by forty percent,[7] an incredible reduction. His success was due to his exceptional ability to make early and accurate diagnoses, his modifications in diets to suit specific illnesses, and his insistence on good hygiene. By the end of 1915 the fall in infant mortality in the hospital had made him famous. Private patients flocked to his office. Baines himself had the grace to recognize Brown's achievement and congratulated the "young whippersnapper" who had been foisted so unceremoniously onto his staff.

After forty years Alan Brown stories still go the rounds, sometimes enriched and magnified by time. As the years pass by, truth can work its way over the edge of reality: "They gave him one of the wards and he started all his various methods of therapy — protein milk (never cow's milk alone) and intravenous or subcutaneous injections of fluids. He cut the mortality by almost one hundred percent. The difference in the two wards was just unbelievable! And when they made him chief the following year or so, he fired the whole medical staff."[8]

The Battle of the Giants

Alan Brown had emerged victorious in his battle with Allen Baines, but with Duncan Graham his fight lasted sixteen years and ended in a standoff.

The year 1919 was the turning point in the careers of both Dr. Alan Brown and another HSC staff member, Dr. Duncan Graham.[9] They received simultaneous appointments. Graham was made chief physician at the Toronto General Hospital and Professor of Medicine at the University of Toronto, while Brown was appointed Physician-in-Chief at the

Hospital for Sick Children but only Associate Professor of Medicine at the University, which placed him under Graham. At HSC their areas of influence were so different that their personalities had little opportunity to clash. Brown's interest and training was focused on the treatment of infants and young children where Graham's inclined to a curriculum of undergraduate and postgraduate research and the care of older children and adults. Although Graham had been senior to Brown at HSC, he had no reason to assert his authority over the younger man and their relationship had remained cordial.

With Graham's top appointment in the Department of Medicine the fat was in the fire, and conflagration inevitable. Graham, as Head of the Department of Medicine, was responsible for assigning the departmental funds.[10] It infuriated Brown that each time he needed funds he had to approach his colleague, cap in hand. He resented Graham's control of the financial allocations to the two teaching hospitals. "Duncan Graham had his own responsibilities at the adult hospital and in adult teaching, but Alan Brown felt he got the short end of the stick. Graham was a strong-minded Scot. Personalities were very, very strong in those days — they had to be because if they weren't they got swept aside."[11]

Thus their feud began. It soon became very bitter indeed. It was a battle of dinosaurs. Each was a strong, stubborn character used to having his own way in life. Each considered the priorities of his own patients and hospital more urgent than the other's. That Bruce Robertson's widow, Enid, married Duncan Graham in 1928 no doubt increased Alan's sense of impotence and hence his dislike of his superior at the University. Repeated collision continued until Alan Brown was made Professor of the new Department of Paediatrics in 1935 when he no longer had to make his financial requests to the University through Duncan Graham.

Chapter 5
Alan Brown's Reign: 1919–1951

Part One — Alan Brown Takes the Helm: The Armistice, The Spanish Influenza Epidemic, The Roaring Twenties, Alan Brown Calls the Shots, Nursing Staff — the Early Years, John Ross Robertson's College Street Hospital

Part Two — Alan Brown's Preventive Medicine: Good Hygiene — His Lasting Legacy, Surgery and Segregation, Nutrition for Infants and Children, Research, Pablum a Winner

Part Three — Clinician and Diagnostician: Rounds and Patient Care, The Stool Pigeon, Clinical Brilliance, Errors and Omissions, Favoured Remedies for "Failure to Thrive"

Part Four — Alan Brown's Hospital: Doctor at Work, Alan Brown amused, The Administrator, Staff Relationships

Part Five — Alan Brown and His Domain: 1929 — 1951: The Great Depression: 1929 — 1939, The Quints, Pasteurization in Ontario, Poliomyelitis, Alan Brown in Demand, The World at War again, Anti-Semitism in the Hospital

Part Six — The Professor and his Students

Part Seven — Conferences, Publications, Plagiarism

Part One — Alan Brown takes the Helm

The Armistice

On the 11th of November 1918 in France at Compiègne, the scene of heavy fighting during the war, the Armistice was signed. A student's diary at the University of Toronto echoes the joy of peace: "At five o'clock this morning I wakened . . . whistles were blowing. . . ."[1] The din rose with increasing enthusiasm as trumpets blared above the beating of drums and the skirl of bagpipes. Impromptu parades were held all across the nation. The diary continues:

> (At) the corner of Yonge and College . . . tens of thousands of marchers passed . . . there were people dressed up in every conceivable costume. . . bonfires. . . confusion. The Sousa band was playing in the park . . . .

As the country awoke, bands began to play everywhere right across the land.

The Spanish Influenza Epidemic

Returning war-weary veterans created the greatest peacetime emergency in Canada's history. They brought home a virulent type of influenza that had infected the troops in Europe during the last days of the fighting. More Canadians sickened and died between 1918 and 1920 than had been killed in four years of battle. Ontario and Quebec alone had over one million cases and twenty thousand deaths. Fear stalked the streets of the nation. In a vain effort to stem the tide, face masks and mothball pendants were worn. Schools and churches emptied, and social events cancelled as the epidemic spread. The diary continues:

> Tuesday, October 15, 1918 . . . all the schools are closed. . . at Varsity classes are dwindling and the professors are going down one by one with the flu. . . . Thursday, October 17 . . . The University will close at one o'clock to-morrow until Tuesday, Nov. 5th if the time is not extended.

Footsteps of skeleton staffs echoed through the government corridors of Queen's Park and City Hall. Domestic chaos reigned. There was no escape for The Hospital for Sick Children as staff and patients equally succumbed. Alan Brown himself fell ill and narrowly escaped death. Another two or three years would have to pass before the worst epidemic in Canadian history was finally exhausted.

In 1923, perhaps caused by the continuing plague of influenza, Alan Brown's close friend Bruce Robertson died of pneumonia. Alan was distraught. He and Connie took the extraordinary step of nursing him in their house: "I always meant to ask mother why Aunt Enid (Robertson) didn't look after Uncle Bruce when he was dying," Alan's daughter Barbara reflected. Alan Bruce-Robertson explains:

> When my father first became ill he was admitted to the TGH. He hated that hospital, so after two or three days Uncle Alan took him home to his Avenue Road house because he had his medical office in the basement and could look after him until he was able to be admitted to the Wellesley where he died. I was only two years old and my sister was a baby. Our parents wanted to protect us from the danger of cross-infection.

The Roaring Twenties
After four years of war followed by the 1918 Spanish influenza epidemic, the Canadian economy was beginning to recover. Toronto's population rose to half a million. Business and professional life returned to peacetime pursuits modified — and enriched — by the experience and demands of war. The city's social set, released from the constraints of war, was impatient to restore a flourishing culture. Theatres and concert halls engaged foreign artists and orchestras: Pavlova in "Swan Lake" at the Royal Alexandra Theatre, Rubinstein, Toscanini and Milan's La Scala at Massey Hall. In 1923 Von Kunits, with the Toronto Symphony Orchestra, conducted the first of his many regular Twilight Symphony concerts in Massey Hall. There was an atmosphere of release and frivolity; Gilbert and Sullivan comic operas played to full houses.

> Everything was different then. There are very few of us left who know anything about the old days when Toronto was so small and meant so much to us. We grew up in the roaring twenties and the twenties really roared, there's no doubt about that — wild parties, bathtub gin and girls going out wearing nothing underneath their evening gowns.[2]

It was the era of the flappers with their bobbed hair, short skirts and bound bosoms: breast feeding became almost extinct. Women craved flat chests so that they could wear the revolutionary new styles. Their short silk dresses were festooned with strings of beads that swayed provocatively on the dance floor. The waltz was out and the Charleston in: "You had to keep pulling down your skirt and hiking up your silk stockings. We weren't blessed with panty hose or nylons in those days." Corsages were put in the ice box until the last moment when they were pinned on the skimpy party frocks, frequently staining or even tearing them. Ironically, men customarily wore white gloves to protect the thin silk dresses from nervously perspiring hands.

Whenever Connie could tear Alan away from his babies, they joined the parties. At their own, Alan made "bathtub gin" as many hosts did in prohibition times. His elder daughter Barbara, then five or six, watched fascinated as her father mixed his concoction. He brought alcohol home from the hospital, dumped it in a large stone crock and proceeded to doctor it with juniper berries, lemons and other ingredients as the spirit moved him. By the time the guests arrived Alan was primed to be an entertaining and jovial host.

Alan Brown Calls the Shots
He had no intention of being diplomatic. Heads rolled after his appointment as Physician-in-Chief of The Hospital for Sick Children in 1919. He fired all the doctors who, in his opinion, had treated children only when it suited them. Of the few he retained at least two of them, Edward Morgan and George Smith, remained on the staff until they retired many years later. Meanwhile, quickly but carefully, he put together a trained and dedicated medical, nursing and research staff.

Thirty-three years old in 1920, Alan Brown exuded enthusiasm and determination. In that year he expanded the number and size of the hospital departments. He recruited Dr. Gladys Boyd,[3] the first woman on the medical staff, to direct endocrine, renal and chest services. In 1921 he set up The Hospital for Sick Children's nutritional laboratories, absolutely crucial to his plans for the development of preventive medicine. The HSC Medical Advisory Board minutes of September 1923 refer to departments of surgery, ophthalmology, laryngology, pathology, bacteriology, anaesthesiology and dentistry. He added substance and depth to medical care. In 1920 he established the first psychological clinic for children in Canada, housed in a YMCA building nearby until space was made available in HSC. He was the first to initiate paediatric divisions of cardiology and neurology. In 1922 he was one of the founders[4] and, in 1923, the second president of The Canadian Society for the Study of Diseases of Children, the early name for The Canadian Paediatric Society.

Nursing Staff — The Early Years
In 1921 Alan Brown turned his attention to his nursing staff and hired the hospital's first Superintendent of Nurses, Miss Kathleen Panton. She was ideally suited to uphold the kind of regimentation and discipline that Alan Brown demanded. Miss Panton had served four years on active service overseas during the war and was accustomed to giving and receiving orders. For the next seventeen years she and her successor, Miss Pearl Austin, "ran that hospital as though they were still in the army".[5] In 1938, Miss Jean Masten, the third Superintendent of Nurses, finally introduced a more humane discipline.

One young applicant to the HSC's School of Nursing remembers Miss Austin with mixed feelings:

> She couldn't have been more charming when she was interviewing me so I signed up for the September class. But once she had my signature her whole attitude changed and she abruptly ordered me out of her office to get measured for a uniform. Stunned but angry I meekly left, went straight home and wrote my resignation letter — certain that life under her would be unbearable. By the time the next class began in February I'd spent all those months in Cobourg with nothing to do but drink and play bridge so I had second thoughts and decided to go to Sick Kids after all.[6]

Upon Miss Panton's retirement Miss Austin became the hospital's second Superintendent of Nurses. Both women were despotic, narrow-minded and their rules archaic, but the discipline they enforced was made to measure for Alan Brown's autocracy. The dress code for nurses during the Roaring Twenties was unbelievable. Within the hospital, the flapper with her skimpy dress riding above her knees certainly did not exist. Nurses were forced to wear ankle-length uniforms with laced black boots, starched, white-bibbed aprons and stiff, fly-away caps perched precariously on their long coiled hair; all this in an era when other young women wore short skirts and cropped heads. No air conditioning cooled the wards in the summer. Nurses sweltered in their heavy long skirts and tightly bibbed shirts as they wrestled with their discomfort. Infringement of the rules brought summary dismissal. Short hair was absolutely forbidden. It was considered frivolous and unprofessional. A nurse who had the temerity to "bob" her hair was immediately dismissed. One probationer successfully hid her cropped head under a wig.[7] By today's standards the rules enforced and the customs followed were not only impractical but absurd. In contrast, the dress of the interns was marginally more comfortable. They could at least undo their jackets on hot days in the wards, always with an eye out ready to button up at the approach of Dr. Alan Brown or his chief resident.

John Ross Robertson's College Street Hospital
In 1918 World War I ended and the hospital lost John Ross Robertson. For more than thirty years he had been a benevolent dictator, the driving force behind the HSC, who used his talents and money to build and equip a children's hospital second to none on the continent. As owner and publisher of *The Evening Telegram* he could appeal to a wide audience for any of the causes he espoused. One of these was the construction of the College Street building which opened its doors in 1892 as the new home for the Sick Kids'. When he died he bequeathed his vast fortune to the hospital on condition its name would not be changed. If this instruction was not followed, the sum involved was to go to The Salvation Army. He understood the appeal of a name's simplicity: The Hospital for Sick Children.

Except for the last few months of his reign as chief physician, Alan Brown's kingdom was located in the same College Street building that, by 1919 and after thirty years of use, was overcrowded, run down, its equipment obsolete. He began to push for a new hospital shortly after he was appointed Physician-in-Chief in 1919. He was frustrated by events: first by the stock market crash of 1929, followed by the Depression of the thirties and finally by World War II. He had to make do with what he had — an antiquated building, chipped bedpans and cockroaches.[8] The demands on the hospital were far too great for its facilities. Working conditions were unacceptable even in those less fastidious days.

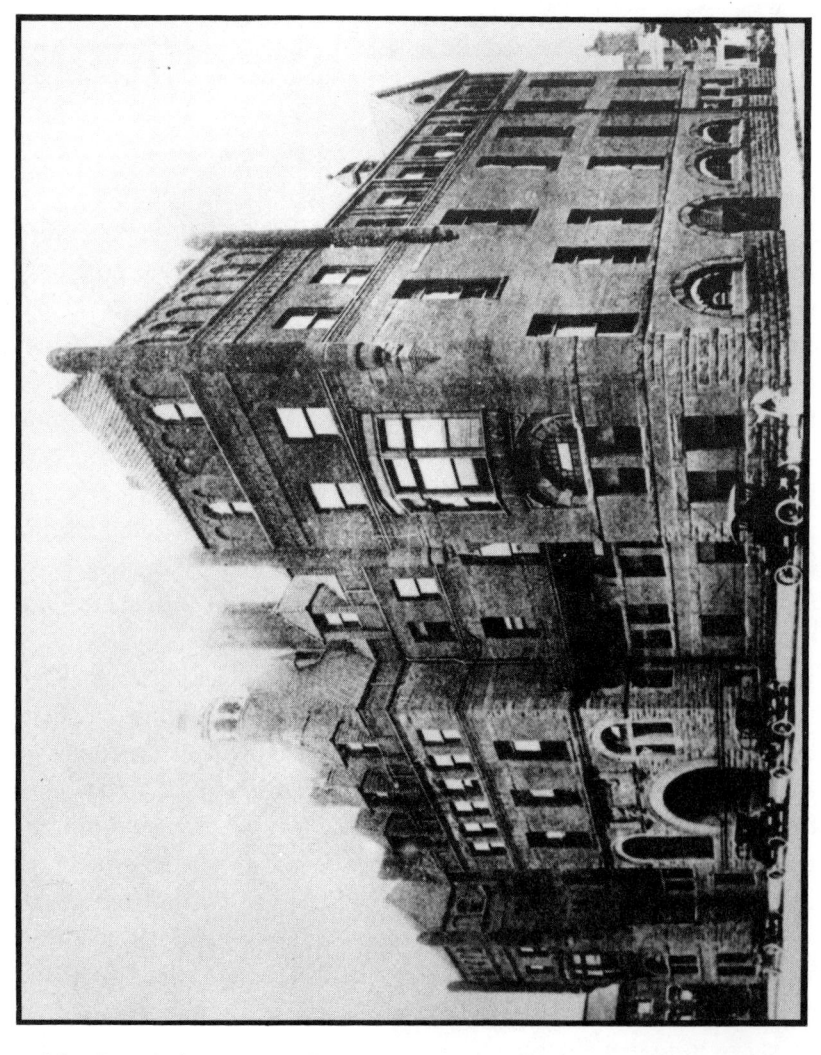

John Ross Robertson's College Street hospital, Toronto. (HSC Archives)

> The Out Patients Department was right opposite the godawful ENT (Ear, Nose and Throat) operating room. Alan used to line up the little kids like jay birds sitting on a bench in the hall waiting to have their tonsils out. They'd haul them in one after the other and you'd hear the suction machines going and the kids yelling. You couldn't help but hear — it was horrible.[9]

Space for female interns in the old hospital's residence was so limited that only two could be appointed at a time.[10] In 1936 Helen Reid from the University of Alberta was accepted, but only after Alan Brown was bombarded by the organized and persistent campaign she waged. Every day he received a letter or a telephone call on her behalf. Amused and exasperated he told Joe Bower, the Superintendant of the hospital, "We'll have to take that Reid woman. I can't stand any more phone calls and letters."[11]

In January 1939, eight months before World War II erupted, Alan Brown appointed the hospital's first female chief resident, Frances Mulligan, gold medallist of her year. Before she could take up her post in July, Dr. Donald McKay, her fiancé, persuaded her that marriage and a chief residency were incompatible. Frances chose marriage and resigned her appointment. No resident had ever before resigned the position and Alan Brown was infuriated by her cheek.

> That wouldn't happen today. We would have handled it differently. Don would never have asked me to give it up. But I have no regrets. There's always more to do in a lifetime than can be done. Every day you have to choose and then make your choices work.[12]

The old College Street hospital's problems may seem amusing now because we are no longer afflicted by them. But some had serious consequences. Cross-infection was a constant concern. There were few ways to control infection in the crowded wards once it had become established; immunization and antibiotics were still in the future. Prevention was the only effective policy. Mice and cockroaches roamed the wards at night. Flies were a source of despair in summer. They invaded the hospital in clouds, thriving on the manure of the nearby Eaton's College Street stables which housed the horsepower for the delivery wagons.

Josephine Kane, one of the hospital's first patients who was allowed to spend most of her life in the nurses' residence, reacted to the annual summer infestation in a naïve but forceful fashion. Exasperated, she wrote to Eaton's complaining that their flies were contaminating the hospital and would they please do something about it. With considerable aplomb, Eaton's replied that they would be delighted to come and collect their flies if Miss Kane would kindly identify them. On another occasion a surgical operation was interrupted while a foraging ant impudently zig-zagged across the instrument table.

The old hospital was so cramped for treatment space that there was scarcely room for visitors, and fears of cross-infection among the babies and children led Alan Brown to impose very strict visiting rules. They seem heartless today but they must be viewed in the context of those times. As one staff physician recalls, "You brought your kid in, almost like dropping off your laundry. The child was examined and sent to a ward and you were sent home." Visiting hours were limited to two to four o'clock on Sundays. But there was no visiting at all in the infectious and infants' wards. A parent then had to climb three flights of a rickety fire escape and peer in the window to try to get a glimpse of the child. The window, covered with grime, obscured the view, which did little to allay the anxiety of the viewer.

The College Street hospital did have its lighthearted moments. The annual Christmas party was a major catalyst. Singing carols, the nurses came slowly down the stairways which wrapped around the old-fashioned elevator. They were accompanied by a piano inside the open elevator which descended slowly from floor to floor at the same pace. Decorated Christmas trees and wreaths with ribbons greeted the VIPs — trustees, clergymen and assorted politicians seated on the main floor to watch the procession and to join in the singing.

Some of the doctors got into the spirit of the season. Bill Mustard, then a surgical intern but later a household name in international paediatric surgery,

> was a pretty little man; short, blond, curly-haired. I remember the year a lovely looking little nurse fell into line with the others. As they sang and walked slowly along past the VIPs she hiked her skirt and winked at Dr. Brown. He was scandalized by her behaviour. Later he was furious he'd been taken in by the

impudent Mustard and took refuge in sarcasm: "too bad we haven't a clown like that on the medical as well as the surgical staff."[13]

The fun and nonsense of the medical students found its outlet in the annual "Daffydil Night", and Dr. Brown was a prime target. At the 1944 performance, he was immortalized in ribald doggerel:

> On the corner of College and Elizabeth, my dears,
> Stands an old red stone building that's been there for years.
> And as you're passing by you may think it absurd
> That voices from inside are frequently heard
> Singing, 'Brown, Brown, dirty old Brown'.
>
> That bombastic old bastard who wears a bow tie,
> Is the doctor described to the folks passing by.
> He's diaper crazy, this stool-happy Brown
> And students will shout till the roof tumbles down
> Singing, 'Brown, Brown, dirty old Brown'.[14]

Four years later:

> For Daffydil Night I had to make a fellow look like Alan Brown for one of the skits. I'd been with Dora Mavor Moore and was pretty good with the greasepaint. This guy Bogoch,[15] had a huge head of curly hair and I had to make him bald without scalping him. I got a silk stocking, greased it all up so it looked like skin and he was one of the best makeups I ever did. This guy really looked just like Alan Brown when I got finished. A banner across the back of the stage read: "Exhibits — Royal Ontario Museum". In the foreground on pedestals like statues we lined up all the profs — Ed. and Gordon Gallie, Roscoe Graham and his cousin Duncan, Alan Brown, Van Wyck and Don Fraser. When the lights came on the audience roared.[16]

During both world wars, the additional duties undertaken by a skeleton staff treating the same number of patients left less time and energy for ribaldry. No one complained about the extra work but it was frustrating to have to struggle against the inadequacies and dangers of the old building. The allocation of funds for the hospital came from a Board of Directors whose decisions were made in the comfortable surroundings of one of their elegant homes. They were not easily persuaded that the old hospital was a civic disgrace and a blot on their reputations. As always, Alan Brown took the direct approach. He decided to change the venue of the Board meeting to the hospital itself. He then asked his chief resident to go through the wards and list all the dangers in the hospital that were beyond repair or remedy:

> We had to have a new hospital. There were cockroaches all over the infectious ward. Mice had a field day in the linen cupboards and flies were everywhere. The trustees arrived. He took them around pointing out all the problems.[17]

The hospital's sorry state shocked the Board into an immediate decision. They promised to build a new hospital as soon as peace was declared. By 1947, in record time and oversubscribed, the funds had been raised. Construction began on University Avenue. Alan Brown, under his yellow hard hat, was often to be seen scrambling over the site relishing the consummation of his dream. He had been pleading for this building for nearly thirty years. His hand had been in everything, at all stages of the planning and construction. His was the inspiration behind the advances and innovations.

Part Two — Alan Brown's Preventive Medicine

Throughout his long medical career Alan Brown repeatedly stressed that "paediatrics is the practice of preventive medicine." Very little could be done for children once they became ill; prevention was imperative.

Good Hygiene — His Lasting Legacy

It is difficult today to realize how fanatical Brown must have seemed to the hospital staff by his insistence on cleanliness. Cleanliness — good hygiene — he used to repeat, was the sheet anchor of preventive medicine. Social cleanliness and tidy wards were not enough for a children's hospital where the smallest slip-up could speed a deadly infection through the building. Isolation and quarantine went hand in hand with good hygiene. Until the sulphonamides appeared in the 1930s there were no antibiotics to rescue a patient population from the ravages that followed sloppy hygiene. Diphtheria spread with deadly effect. (Although diphtheria antitoxin had been developed in the early years of the twentieth century, its impurity often caused severe reactions.)

> He was known to have fired a nurse who neglected to change a dirty diaper. After that incident a nurse always followed him on rounds with a clean diaper at the ready tucked behind her back. If it was unexpectedly needed as Dr. Brown approached, she was ready to say, "Oh, Dr. Brown! I was just going to change it."[18]

Brown's finicky hygienic obsessions reached right down to any errant dust ball that might have gathered under a cot. He was forever on the watch for infractions of his hygiene regulations. Whenever he had time between his morning rounds and his lecture at noon he would check around the hospital to make sure all was as it should be.

> He would walk through Outpatients where the mothers would be waiting, their babies often sucking on little nippled soothers. These he would gently remove and throw into the nearest garbage can. He was oblivious to the wailing that followed.[19]

Seventy years later it is still difficult to keep up to Alan Brown's high standards. During the summer of 1990 a University of Toronto graduate student, Sari Weinberg, decided to write her thesis on the quality of hygiene on two wards in HSC. In one she observed careful attention to achieve constant cleanliness and in the other the attention was neither careful nor constant. The results of her research were not surprising. There was far less cross-infection in the first ward, more pride in the care of the patients and a higher recovery rate. The breakdown of cleanliness routines in the second ward may have been encouraged by the staff's over-dependence on antibiotics for the prevention and cure of infections.

Surgery and Segregation
One of Alan Brown's battle cries was, "Find the focus of infection and remove it." This principle was and is orthodox. Brown based his treatment on zealous application of the principle. Infected teeth and tonsils

were the usual culprits. Streptococcus and staphylococcus infections were common in the mouth and throat, and teeth and tonsils were easy to remove. Without the prophylactic protection of antibiotics it is probable that at least some children were harmed by operations by dislodging bacteria at the infected site into the blood stream. A common focus of infection was the middle ear, Laurie Chute chuckles:

> As an intern, before Alan Brown made his rounds on my ward, I would go to two or three cases with puzzling fevers and even if the otoscope showed nothing I would sometimes puncture an ear just in case it was infected. I had to check all possibilities before he came along.

When, in spite of good nutrition, a child failed to thrive, Dr. Brown would invariably order the tonsils to be removed. Dr. Charles Best was well aware of the danger of cross-infection in a hospital:

> When his son Henry had a tonsillectomy, he was barely off the operating table before his father scooped him up and ran down the stairs hotly pursued by Alan shouting, "You can't do this, Charlie. Looks bad for the hospital." Dr. Best yelled over his shoulder as he ran out of the hospital, "I most certainly can. I'm not going to leave him here to pick up ten other infections!"[20]

Nutrition for Infants and Children
In 1911, while Brown was studying in New York, an essential step in preventive medicine was taken by Dr. Charles Hastings, Toronto's first Medical Officer in its new Department of Health. He persuaded the city fathers to legislate the enforcement of pasteurization of milk in the city.[21] To have pasteurized milk readily available for the Hospital for Sick Children's "milk lab" saved Alan Brown a great deal of time and effort when he prescribed lactic acid and protein milks. The result of the legislation was dramatic. Almost immediately it reduced the incidence of tuberculosis. But the disease continued unabated among those from out of town until 1935. In that year Alan Brown persuaded the premier of Ontario, Mitchell Hepburn, to pass legislation that would compel the province's farmers to bear the cost of pasteurization before the milk left the farm — a politically and personally difficult undertaking because he was a farmer himself elected by a farming constituency.

The changes Brown made in patient care and treatment, particularly in diets, were profound. Special diets to suit every condition were introduced: for example, lactic acid milk for celiacs, rice cereal and protein milk for infant diarrheas supplemented with intravenous fluids to correct dehydration.

> The special feedings — they were really what made him famous. Every formula was worked out to the last detail. We had a nurse who sat in a little back room and plotted the graph on each baby's chart to show the proportion of fat and protein and carbohydrate in the formula. He got a lot of ridicule when he first came. They referred to him as "that dietician."[22]

> He called protein milk "the sheet anchor of infant feeding" because it would cure so many of the children with chronic diarrhea from various causes of which many, such as lactose intolerance, were not even identifed at that time. But his methods were curing the children; why, we didn't know.[23]

Research

In 1920 Brown persuaded Miss Angelia Courtney, a Radcliffe graduate, to leave New York and come to Toronto to direct the hospital's new chemical research laboratories — the Nutritional Research Laboratories, as he preferred to call them. In addition, she was to oversee the "milk lab" which prepared the protein and lactic acid milks, butter soups and the other special formulas that he prescribed. He had been impressed with her research when he was a resident at the Babies' Hospital in New York; he had written a couple of medical papers with her. He wanted her, with her special knowledge, to support his clinical work, to develop products containing the ingredients that would give children enriched and balanced diets and to make up special formulas for children with metabolic disorders.

Pablum a Winner. Gruel out the Window

When, in 1929, Miss Courtney resigned as director of HSC's Nutritional Research Laboratories, Alan Brown appointed Drs. F.F. Tisdall and T.G.H. Drake to widen the benefit of the hospital's research to the public. They persuaded dairies and bakeries to add vitamin D to their milk and bread products to eliminate rickets which was still common in children who lacked dietary vitamin D. Pablum[24] and Sunwheat biscuits were two commercially successful creations of Sick Kids' research labs.

Many believe that the formulation and success of Pablum was entirely the product of Brown's knowledge and ingenuity channelled, at his direction, through the special skills of Tisdall and Drake. Dr. Nelles Silverthorne thinks the idea was Tisdall's. Dr. Fred Weinberg's recollection, however, is that although Brown and Tisdall got the credit, the original Pablum formula was in Drake's handwriting. Dr. Drake's widow, Nina, is emphatic that Alan hadn't anything to do with Pablum, an assertion strongly denied by Brown's grandson, Tim Kelley. Tim states that his grandfather told Tisdall and Drake what he wanted in it and they made it up for him.

Tim Kelley may be closer to the truth than Nina Drake. The whole thrust of Alan Brown's preventive medicine was proper diet. During the decade before the development of Pablum, Tim's grandfather was continuously experimenting with various formulas to produce an edible but nutritious hot cereal with a balance of grains and proteins reinforced with vitamins and minerals. He ordered these ever-changing but unappetizing formulas to be given to the ward patients. He also inflicted the gruel on his private patients. Over the years, hundreds of mothers and children suffered from the birth pangs of Pablum. Alan Brown's gruel became notorious — to be avoided at all costs. After one or two attempts at force-feeding, many of his most faithful mothers refused to inflict it on their offspring. The hospital's patients had no choice.

One young mother of four little boys, terrified into obedience, religiously followed the diet Alan Brown had ordered. Every night at six o'clock they were sent to their bedrooms and their supper, the infamous gruel, was brought up to them. Rather than go to bed hungry they forced some of it down until one of them hit on the idea of stealing cakes and cookies their mother kept in a locked kitchen cupboard. They unscrewed the hinges, selected the forbidden items as their emergency rations for that night and dispatched the gruel through the bedroom window. This arrangement worked well until spring when a dirty gray "stucco" was discovered on the red brick wall below the third-floor window.

The painstaking persistence of the HSC Nutritional Research Laboratories paid off. In 1935 Tisdall set up the Paediatric Research Foundation "to receive the royalties from Pablum and Sunwheat biscuits. The income was soon large enough to supply all the instruments and equipment for our research lab."[25] Nearly twenty years later the Foundation turned over $1,700,000 to the HSC Research Institute which had been incorporated in 1951. From the days of the milk lab, completed in 1913, through Alan Brown's Nutritional Research Laboratories, first directed by Miss Courtney and later expanded by Tisdall and his assistant director, Drake, nutritional research at Sick Kids' has flourished. Alan Brown, with the stress he placed on nutrition as an important part of preventive medicine, had finally won for it the serious attention he knew it deserved.

Part Three — Clinician and Diagnostician

Rounds and Patient Care

Anyone who did not follow Alan Brown's orders or who was indifferent or careless was fired. Whether he had the right to do this or not, didn't matter; he did it. As Physician-in-Chief he did not hesitate to shoulder total responsibility for maintaining the high standards he had set, whether they concerned patients' medical treatment, hygienic procedures, nutrition and special diets, his student lectures in paediatrics or the administration of the hospital.

His hospital day began at seven. The chief resident would be waiting for him in his office. In 1933 Bill Hawke, holding this precarious position, had worked out a fool-proof warning system with Mrs. Groves, the switchboard operator who sat just inside the College Street door. "She could spot Alan's mood when he arrived. We had arranged a signal. I'd get a quick call from her, either 'Storm warning' or 'Sunny day ahead'. This worked like a charm." After the briefing by his chief resident, Alan Brown began his day with ward rounds.

Ten years later the hospital's loudspeaker alerted another chief resident:

> "Dr. Sugarman, Dr. Sugarman, Dr. Brown is in." I didn't like getting up early so I'd still be dashing through the wards to hear what had come in the night before — they'd hand me a cup of coffee as I flew by — then after the intercom's warning I'd rush to meet him in his office. If I fumbled a question, he'd say, "You live here and you don't know what's going on?" You had to know ALL about the four hundred patients, a dozen of whom might have come in the night before. Then, after informing him about the new patients and developments, I'd escort him on the morning's rounds.

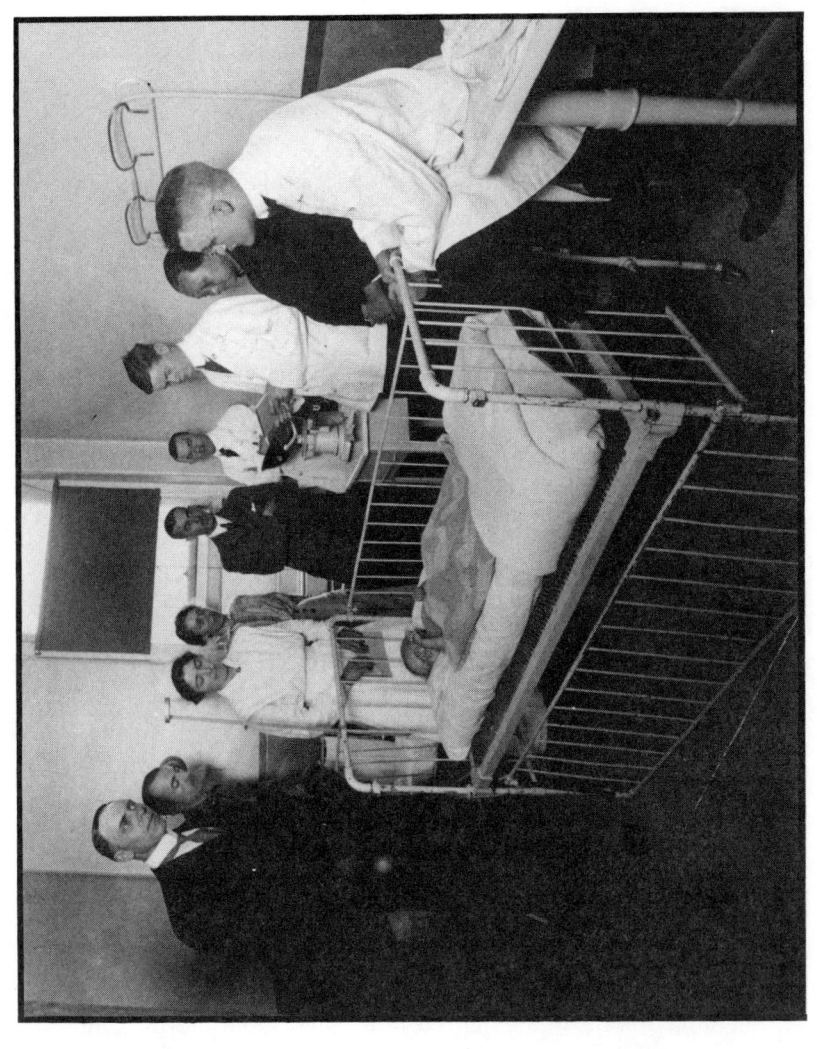

Alan Brown (on the right) on ward rounds with visiting doctors in the early 1920s (HSC Archives)

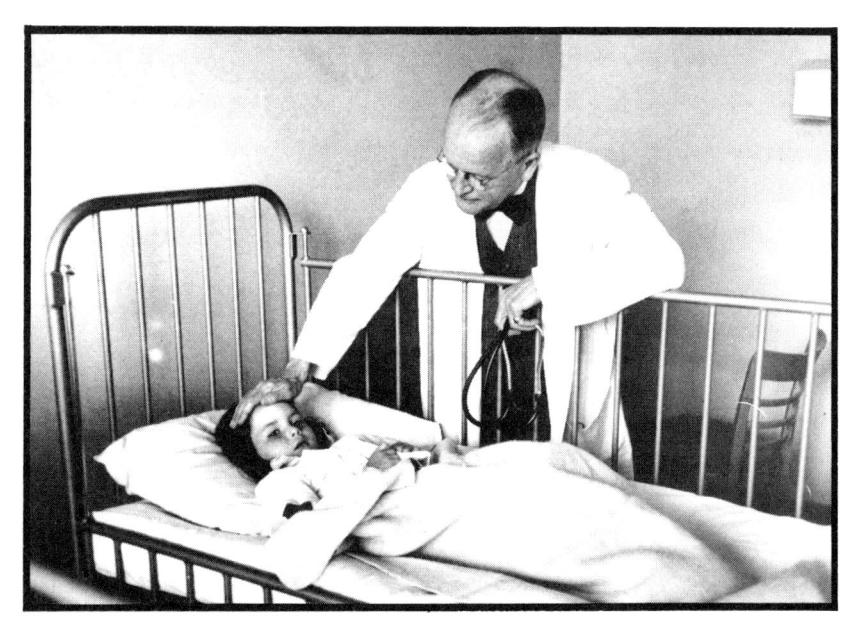

Alan Brown comforts a patient (photo H.W. Tetlow, Courtesy Maclean's Magazine)

Twice a week "rounds" included all the medical staff, but on these occasions the staff assembled in the lecture hall rather than on the wards. At Grand Rounds, as they were (and still are) called, the medical staff had to sign in before the door was locked at nine o'clock.

Justin (Gus) O'Brien, the last chief resident to serve a full term under Alan Brown, passed his first seven months in the old College Street Hospital and the last five in the new building on University Avenue:

> When he arrived we would first check the black book which listed every patient admitted to the hospital in the past twenty-four hours. He would bark questions, make comments and criticisms before we set off to examine them. Followed by other residents and several nurses, we would then make our way from bed to bed, discussing diagnoses and treatments. He made notes on the patients' charts and demonstrated his clinical skills to the young doctors.

Bernard Laski adds:

> After ward rounds we would all go to the lecture hall to discuss the cases we'd seen. He would sit inside the door with his little notebook where he would write something every time someone came in late. He didn't say anything and we never knew what he wrote. It was intimidating.

The Stool Pigeon
In the days before effective medication and immunization, it was specially important to "read" a baby's stools as an aid to diagnosis and to monitor the course of an intestinal illness. Brown took his residents on stool rounds every morning. The dirty diaper would be placed at the foot of each cot to await the arrival of Brown and his entourage. The odour, the appearance and the shape of the stools were essential clues to diagnosis. "Stools can tell you everything about a baby — except its name," was one of his favourite aphorisms. When a fresh specimen of a particular condition could not be obtained he would pull from his pocket an imitation stool he had brought back from Germany for teaching, or one he had requested the hospital's pathology department to make for him.

Clinical Brilliance

A man must be judged in the context of his times. Alan Brown was primarily a clinician and a teacher in an era when teaching a specialty was new. His great achievement was his ability to pass on skills that were vital at that time. Diagnosis was personal then, a product of the examiner's senses — touch, sight, hearing and smell. The lab was secondary. Today it is paramount; a diagnosis is seldom decided without information that only the laboratory and special investigation can supply.

Alan Brown's brilliance was dimmed by the advent of antibiotics — the sulphonamides in the 1930s and penicillin administered from 1945 at HSC[26] — and by the increasing accuracy of lab tests which have reduced the pre-eminence of clinical skills in diagnosis but will never entirely supersede them. Brown's diagnostic acumen was justifiably renowned: "He could just look at a baby and he'd know what was wrong. Laurie (Chute) would arrive at the same diagnosis but only after a careful examination," Chute's wife, Dr. Helen Reid, observes. Time and time again his perceptive eye and his sensitive fingertips gave him the correct diagnosis. Often quick action was critical for effective treatment. Bill Hawke gives an example:

> On one occasion a child who had been in a motor accident arrived in Emergency. We were trying to diagnose the injuries when Alan came along and after a quick examination said, "He's got a ruptured spleen." He was an excellent diagnostician. (Immediate surgery saved the child's life.)

As head of neurology and the fledgling department of psychiatry, Dr. W.A. Hawke was lecturing to a group of American neurologists while he led them through the wards. There was a child in the infants' ward who just did not seem to be developing the way he should. Hawke described all the tests they had done but the diagnosis remained elusive. At that point Alan Brown arrived and was introduced to the group. As he walked up to the bed he said, "Give me an opthalmoscope." He looked into the boy's eyes and pronounced: "Well, Dr. Hawke, there's your diagnosis: Tay-Sachs disease." The cherry red spot on the retina was the diagnostic point. Alan Brown would repeatedly produce the correct diagnosis when others were puzzled. He thrived on his clinical acuity. He never opened his mouth unless he was sure. But he was not always right.

Errors and Omissions

Alan Brown found it difficult to face the fact that he could make a mistake.

> When he did, he would try to ignore it or wriggle around it somehow. He always thought he was right. He'd probably know when he was wrong but I don't think he'd give in. He wouldn't admit it.[27]

Bill Hawke, who knew him well, never saw Alan back down. As Physician-in-Chief and Professor of Paediatrics he felt he could not allow his medical judgement to be questioned. He had to keep the upper hand. He would accept the assistance of another opinion but once he had made a diagnosis he would not change his mind. Consultation was not his way. He did not consult anyone. Once he had made up his mind he stuck with his decision, even when the evidence was against him. Bernie Laski observed this failing soon after being appointed in 1948 to a junior position:

> I can remember one time when he wouldn't admit he was wrong. Even then medical knowledge was doubling every ten years and he had started to fall behind. No one can keep up. Well, Alan Brown didn't believe in cystic fibrosis. At that time it was just beginning to be recognized. It's a disease of children in which the sweat and mucous glands do not function properly and the lungs and pancreas are affected. I had a patient with cystic fibrosis. I'd made the diagnosis and told the parents the grim outlook; it's bad enough now but it was hopeless then. They wanted Alan Brown in consultation. He came, looked at the child and said, "That's coeliac disease, he'll be alright." He told the parents to give the infant one of his special diets. We followed his treatment. About three months later the kid was in terrible shape. Again Dr. Brown was consulted and again he predicted that the child had coeliac disease and would eventually get better. The child died. In the end he may have believed my diagnosis, but he was stubborn: he wouldn't admit it. All the same, I was one of the few who liked him; I really did. I was grateful for his help.

During the many years they worked together at the HSC, Bill Hawke and Alan Brown circled each other like boxers in the ring. Hawke could seldom win a round even when he was right:

> One day the nurse at my son's school rang to say that he had a fever with stomach pains and nausea. I picked him up and took him down to Alan who X-rayed him with his office fluoroscope. He said, "Oh, there's nothing wrong with him. Go home and have your wife give him an enema." But I was convinced he had appendicitis. I took him down to the hospital. A diseased appendix was removed. When I told Alan he said, "Oh no! It couldn't have been," because he hadn't seen anything on his bloody little X-ray screen — not that it would have shown the appendix anyway. He even refused to go to the lab to see the specimen. This was really ironic, for Alan was known for whipping out the appendix of almost any kid with abdominal pain.

Not everyone agreed that he would never acknowledge his errors. Some of his medical and nursing colleagues came to the rescue of his reputation to assert that Alan Brown was a big enough man to admit his mistakes, at least to himself. At home he might chuckle when he found he was wrong but he felt he couldn't afford to admit any errors at the hospital.

On one occasion, the findings at an autopsy forced him to concede his error. Jack Slavens recalls:

> I'd diagnosed congenital cystic kidneys in a newborn with huge swollen ankles. Years before, at the Mayo Clinic, I had seen a similar case, so I sent this one to Brown's attention at Sick Kids. The baby was in for a week and then he sent it home. He called me, "We couldn't confirm your diagnosis." About a week later the kid's swelling increased so I sent it in again. This time it died. They always die because they have no kidneys — just cysts. After the autopsy he 'phoned me: "You were right," he admitted.

Favoured Remedies for "Failure to Thrive"
Brown had three fads he never gave up: thyroid deficiency, infected tonsils and inflamed appendix. Any child who failed to develop at the normal rate was given thyroid extract, although the cause of slow growth was often simply a normal delay in the maturation process.

He used his office fluoroscope constantly, as much to dazzle as to diagnose. It was a great ally, reinforcing a mother's belief that he was superior to other paediatricians. Fred Weinberg explained:

> He would fluoroscope the kid and if, for example, he saw gaseous distention of the bowel, he would diagnose coeliac disease even though the diagnosis could not be made on that criterion alone. It would look as though the other paediatrician or physician who saw the kid had missed it. It was a kind of showmanship. You put the lights out and the mother and kid are standing there in the dark and can see the image. Nobody else did that in his office.

If he decided an appendectomy or tonsillectomy was indicated, he would call for one of the "plumbers", as he scornfully referred to "his" surgeons. Eddy Robertson was the only one he valued, perhaps because he never questioned Alan Brown's diagnoses and operated on demand. Brown and Wishart, the senior ear, nose and throat surgeon, rubbed one another the wrong way. "They were very much alike — both pompous — and Dr. Wishart was another perfectionist — in his work and in his appearance."[28] When Wishart refused to operate on one of Alan Brown's patients slated for tonsillectomy, their relationship was further strained. Phyllis Norton, RN, in charge of the ear, nose and throat operating room for many years had often seen the clash of their personalities: Wishart had his own ideas and it was not likely he would agree with anything his colleague suggested.

There was another surgeon who resisted Brown's demands. William S. Keith never got along with Brown after he had refused Brown's instruction to remove an appendix. Their relationship had never been easy.

> Bill Keith was the kind who threw things when he got mad. I didn't like a doctor who did that — but he was very clever. One day he came into Alan Brown's office. He didn't bow and scrape to Alan as some of them did. He just went in. "I have a problem. You have a young smart alec on your intern staff by the name of Bill Mustard. He is going to create chaos in this hospital." (Bill Mustard was lots of fun, you know. He used to get tight; nobody knew it but we did, so when he came into the

He didn't say a word. Soon afterwards Mother and Father were chaperones at a hospital party at the Hunt Club. The next morning at rounds, Dad whispered out of the corner of his mouth and with a twinkle in his eye, "Miss Boxhill, why didn't I see you at the dance last night?"

The Administrator

Administration was another of Brown's talents. He was superb. He could grasp the whole picture and all the details that went into its production. Impressed by the smooth-running dictatorships of Dr. Emmett Holt at the Babies' Hospital in New York and the brilliant but imperious professors who taught him in Europe, Brown himself set out on his studied career of autocracy. He noted his mentors never said, "I don't know," or "I'll find out." Those phrases were not a part of their vocabulary. They always had the answer and their confidence never wavered. He modelled his persona on theirs and did not try to conceal his delight in the role of dictator. He played it for thirty-six years, first when he was on trial as physician in charge of an infants' ward in 1915, then as chief physician until he retired in 1951. Even so, he had an uphill battle to get his ideas across. He had to be ruthless when the staff neglected to follow his orders.

During the last twenty-two years of his long reign he found an ally in Joseph Bower, a civil engineer who had supervised the building of Toronto's handsome Union Station on Front Street. In 1928 he was appointed Superintendent of The Hospital for Sick Children to assist Alan Brown with its administration and to oversee the building of the proposed new hospital. Joe was handsome, intelligent and popular, a smooth administrator in contrast to Brown's abrasive supervision. They complemented each other effectively in the management of the hospital. Both men were satisfied with perfection. Not a day went by but Alan would drop into Joe's office. He relied on Joe's persuasion when his own intolerance had ended in stalemate. Joe was patient in his handling of senior staff and employees, but patience wasn't always enough in his dealings with Alan Brown; a certain amount of cunning was sometimes needed.

There was a staff doctor Brown didn't like very much. He said to Joe, "We can't have him here. Get rid of him." Joe did nothing, waiting for his opportunity. A week or so later the man's name came up again but in another context. "Last week," said Joe to Alan, "you said we'd have to keep McCreary on staff, but don't you think we should get rid of him?" "Oh no! We'll keep him on." Joe knew he could rely on Alan's adverse reaction to any suggestion not his own.

Brown usually held the Board of Trustees in the palm of his hand, but on one occasion the Board balked. It voted against allocating funds to enlarge the convalescent hospital at Thistletown. When Joe reported this decision to him, Alan blew up. "Fire the damn Board! I'll tell Bobby Laidlaw (Chairman) to get another Board!" The Board remained intact but, once again, Alan Brown got his way and funding was assured.

During the thirty-two years he was Physician-in-Chief at the Hospital and Professor of Paediatrics at the University he did not receive a salary from either institution. In comparison, Dr. Nelles Silverthorne was paid $700 for his 1927-8 fellowship as a junior member of the staff, and even interns were given a pittance. Alan's private practice supported all his efforts in the hospital including those as the University lecturer in paediatrics. He retired without any pension from either the hospital or the university, having supplemented from his own resources the annual grant of $800 allocated for any extra expenses in the running of the paediatric department. For example, he paid out of his own pocket for books and journals he contributed to the small hospital library. He felt personally and financially responsible for the effective operation of The Hospital for Sick Children.

Staff Relationships

Alan Brown was as demanding of himself as he was of his nursing and medical staff. He was contented in his autocratic role and pleased with the results. But even those who were fond of him knew him to be a bully. Here's what some of his colleagues thought of him:

- He thought he ran a tight ship in the right direction — He didn't think he was a bully.
- He didn't like yes-men. He liked strong personalities.
- He bullied those who were meek and mild, even if they were doing a good job.
- You had to be ready to stand up to Dr. Brown.
- He played a cat-and-mouse game — he'd try to corner you with his questions. You had to anticipate them.

- He certainly made life miserable for Hal Edwards, a fine paediatrician but too slow to satisfy Alan.
- Alan used to make Hal's wife miserable too. She used to get physically ill when he came on her ward. She'd try to slip out if she could. She was terrified.
- When I went in as a resident I was scared stiff. I'd heard so many stories about him.
- He was abrupt and he was rude. He made terrible comments that really hurt.
- He was a horrid little man.

In spite of such outspoken opinions there were those who liked him immensely. Almost everyone who had the opportunity to work closely with him, including some of the staff quoted, not only had great respect for his ability but found they had developed a real affection for him. Even the last blunt opinion was tempered by a pardoning afterthought: "Maybe his tactics were necessary at that time." Some of them certainly were. Helen McCallum remembers:

> Many interns and residents arrived full of self-importance; they had more of it than they were ever going to need for the rest of their lives. They'd snap orders at the nurses and wouldn't listen if we tried to tell them something. And it was difficult to get them out of bed at night to attend to a very sick child. Their priorities were often out of whack. Small wonder that Alan Brown pounced on them. He would bark "Always listen to the nurses; you can learn a lot from them." I don't know any other doctors who did that — perhaps John Keith, Dr. Goldbloom.

He was always considerate of the nurses — except Florence Edwards. She was so intimidated by him she couldn't think straight; her mind closed down when he came near her. All the nurses were wary of him but many were prepared to defend their actions. The uneasy atmosphere he created in the hospital kept his staff alert and efficient if not always good-tempered. As Bernie Laski described it:

> He'd fire some of them repeatedly — Sandy Goodchild, Pete Snelling — good paediatricians who lost their hospital privileges

frequently. I'm not sure he ever fired Bill Hawke but there was friction between them. "Who's next?" was the question bantered around the hospital. Sometimes his staff struck back and actually won the odd round. In the staff room Alan Brown used to post the names of those who were delinquent. One day somebody put Brown's name down with the comment, COULD DO BETTER. He was furious but was unable to find out who did it.

Rarely were his orders defied. Theo Drake was a workaholic and just as obstinate as Alan. He was engrossed by his research and he could not tolerate interruptions:

> Alan wanted to bring Lady Eaton and some other VIPs up to the lab. He ordered Theo: "I want all your staff to wear clean lab coats and to line up in the corridor." Theo retorted, "My staff are here to work, not to be on display. Their lab coats will be in their usual state of disarray and my staff will not line up to curtsey to anybody."

Friction between the two men resulted in a rare apology from Alan Brown:

> One day Theo came up to the lab. He said nothing but was white with anger. He did not look at me. Then the phone rang and I heard him reply, "It's all right, Sir, don't worry about it." Alan was phoning to apologize — incredible! I was dying to know why, but I never found out. Theo refused to tell me.

To avoid a crushing reprimand or even dismissal for an error or oversight, you had to recognize your mistake before he did:

> — One of his lads, a resident, Joe Jackson, a big, jolly chap, transfused a child with the wrong blood type. Immediately he realized his error and was as upset as hell. He woke me up — it was about two or three o'clock in the morning. I knew that when Alan came in next day and found out what had happened the roof would blow off. He would have kicked Joe out of the hospital. He had the power to do it — at least nobody had the power to tell him he didn't. There was only

one thing to do. We woke Alan up and told him the story: "We thought you should know this without delay. We are watching the child closely and so far there are no ill effects." Nothing happened. There was no explosion from Alan because Joe had admitted it. But if Alan had arrived in the morning and hadn't been warned about the mistake all hell would have broken loose when he found out.[33]

— The first time I was on days — in Girls' Medical — he appeared in the ward. I don't know where the head nurse was but there he was and there was I, scared to death. As I escorted him down the ward toward his patient he suddenly turned to me and said, "Have you been to Europe?" I replied, "No, I haven't." "Well," he said, "if you go, you'll find out that the hospitals over there look just like this," and he pointed to some fluff under the beds. "Why," I said "this is disgraceful — I'll see that it's swept up right away." That's the only time I was afraid I was in for a blast. If you stood up to him, then everything was fine. He tested people. He was a little short man and a bully. A lot of small men try to compensate in this way. If he was able to push you around he wouldn't have much use for you afterwards.[34]

The attending medical staff had to work three hours a day for four days a week in the Out Patients' Department for the privilege of being on the Sick Kids' staff. Some, such as Frank Park and Gordon Manace, whose priority was private practice, were fired. Manace tried to save face with a resignation letter. In it he wrote, "My time at the Sick Kids has been both arduous and unpleasant."[35] One of his contemporaries, Jack Slavens, bluntly damned him. "He was bounced, fired. He was incompetent and lazy, but he told everyone he'd resigned because he couldn't stand Alan Brown."

Hal Edwards found working with Alan Brown difficult. He eventually resigned to become chief of paediatrics at the Scarborough General Hospital. Another distinguished paediatrician was lost to Sick Kids' for the same reason; when the Childrens' Hospital of Eastern Ontario in Ottawa asked him to take over as chief of medicine, Jack Fletcher accepted.

One senior resident remembers the ups and downs of his year with Alan Brown:

The year I spent as his houseman was the highlight of my life, but our relationship had a rough beginning. Checking through the wards one day I found out a doctor had given a verbal order instead of writing it down in detail. He had told a nurse to slap a mustard plaster on a baby. The baby got badly burned. I decided not to report him but to give him hell myself. But on rounds the next day one of the nurses told Dr. Brown. Furious, he turned on me, "McGarry, you're hiding behind this nurse's skirts." I turned my back and walked off the ward, wrote out my resignation and took it down to Mr. Bower's office. I was barely back in the houseman's quarters when I got a call from the office. Dr. Brown had gone in to see what was new and Mr. Bower had handed him my resignation. When I arrived they both looked at me.

"McGarry, did you write this?"

"Yes, I've had enough."

"Oh now, I didn't really mean what I said. I was just mad at what happened. It wasn't your fault."

"I know that . . .that's why I'm resigning."

Grumpily, but as close to smiling as he ever got, he said, "Take this away and tear it up."

From that moment we got along beautifully. Even so, I carried the resignation in my pocket for the rest of my residency. I never used it again but I was tempted a couple of times. When I was leaving the hospital to go into practice he gave me a good piece of advice: "Don't be afraid to get a consultation, or two or three. If you're right it will add to your reputation and confidence." To this day I still use the printed instructions he gave the nursing mothers.

Without exception, residents and junior staff who worked closely with Alan Brown found him exacting but fair. Their respect for him cannot be doubted. It remains fresh in their memories to this day.

Brown had no compunction about dismissing those who did not live up to the high standards he set for himself and his staff. He fired at least five staff doctors who consistently made house calls instead of honouring their commitment to the teaching of medical students. "He put them on the spot. 'Either you teach or you get out.' They got out."

There was great prestige but no financial reward in a hospital appointment. Some doctors felt they could not afford to give unpaid time when family responsibilities demanded the income from a full-time private practice. Others, a minority, simply preferred the indulgence of a large income to satisfy their material tastes.

Alan Brown did not play favourites. "Even though John Oille was Dad's doctor at TGH, he fired his intern son after bawling him out." Nor could he tolerate incompetence, carelessness or indifference. But a few offenders were given a second chance. During World War II, according to Bob Farber, there was a resident who

> was terrible, really incompetent. Since we were short-staffed, it was not until he became dangerous that Alan Brown fired him. Eventually he even lost his licence to practise.

In one instance, against his better judgement, Alan Brown had to put up with an intern's absent-minded negligence. Lilian Clark is still indignant:

> This one was absolutely hopeless, one of the worst we ever had. He'd leave his ward unattended or stand in a daze looking out the window, forgetting his duties. He was madly in love and would dash off the minute she rang or appeared. He was bright enough but completely irresponsible. Alan Brown asked me, "Is he really doing all these things?" "Yes, indeed he is," I replied. He was furious, but reluctantly concluded, "Well, we'll have to keep him on. We can't let him go." His family had contributed a lot of money to the hospital. "You'll have to cover for him." And I did. But he wasn't back the next year, I'll tell you that!

Part Five — Alan Brown and His Domain: 1929-1951

The Great Depression, 1929-1939

After the stock market crash of '29, the Roaring Twenties imploded and the Great Depression of the thirties took over. The contrast in life styles between the rich and the poor was accentuated. Debutante parties and the trappings of launching young women into society contrasted cruelly with the dispirited clusters of the unemployed lining up at soup kitchens. There was no health or unemployment insurance and no government

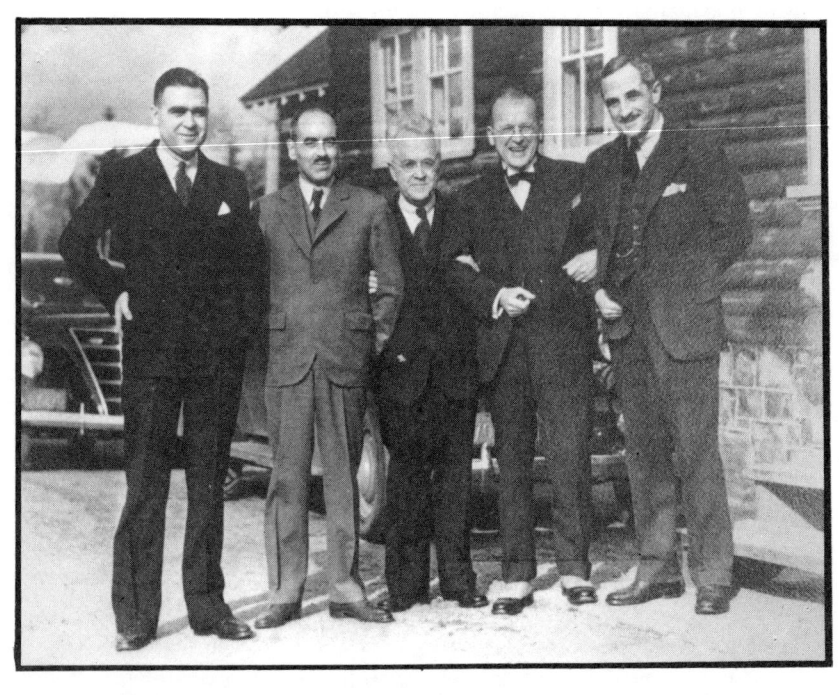

1938: treatment team for the Dionne quintuplets' tonsillectomy: Drs. J.F. McCreary, C.H. Robson, Allan Dafoe, Alan Brown and D.E.S. Wishart (HSC Archives)

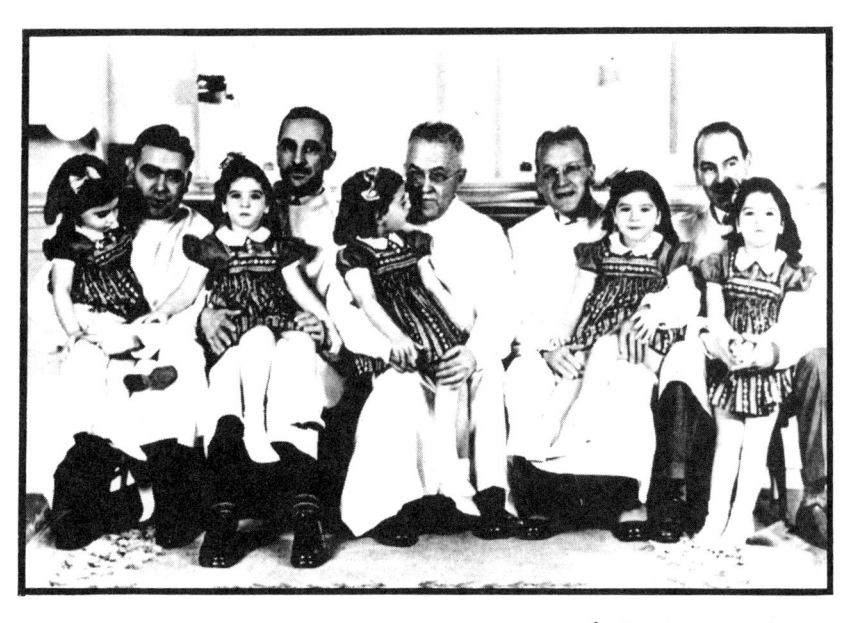

The same five with the famous five: Annette, Cécile, Émilie, Marie and Yvonne (HSC Archives)

welfare cheques to ease the pain. Men rode the rails across the country seeking work. Meanwhile, medicine leaped into its future role as vaccines and sulpha drugs began to contain the scourge of viral and bacterial epidemics.

During the Depression, Alan Brown and his hospital were involved in three major events: the birth of the world's first quintuplets, pasteurization of milk throughout Ontario, and the polio epidemic.

The Quints

On the twenty-eighth of May 1934 the Dionne quintuplets were born at home, in a log cabin without electricity or plumbing, on the outskirts of the village of Corbeil near Callander in northern Ontario. They were the first quintuplets in the world to survive. Their successful arrival was due to the skill of Dr. Allan Dafoe, the Dionne's family doctor. Their combined weight was about twelve pounds — one-and-a-half to two-and-a-half pounds each. Five tiny bodies with arms and legs the size of their parents' fingers. Their continuing survival was largely due to the paediatric training, experience and determined interference of Dr. Alan Brown and his staff. He was in daily contact with Dr. Dafoe and he periodically sent his chief resident, Jack McCreary, to ensure adherence to the strict hygienic and dietetic regimen he had prescribed. As a further precaution, he persuaded the Government of Ontario to make the babies wards of the province.[36]

> Many objected to taking them away from their parents but they would otherwise have died. As soon as they were born, the babies were carefully wrapped in a blanket and put in a clothes basket placed at the door of the open oven to keep them warm. It was really a miracle they lived. We didn't have intravenous therapy or anything like that for them. If Dr. Brown hadn't been able to have them isolated hygienically and fed properly they wouldn't have survived.[37]

Their father, Oliva Dionne, showed no warmth towards his famous little girls. He treated them as a business asset and actually signed a contract to exhibit his babies at the Chicago World's Fair, alongside, no doubt, the fat lady and other unfortunate freaks of nature. At that point the province heeded Alan Brown's advice and removed the Quints from their parents, a move facilitated, we may assume, by Brown's acquaintance with his surgical colleague Herbert Bruce, Lieutenant-Governor of Ontario.

Dionne's mercenary instincts were offensive:

> When my sister was quite young, Dad asked Mr. Dionne, "Would you autograph this photograph of your babies for my little girl?" The father of the Quints, not hesitating for a moment, replied, "There are signed copies you can buy over there at the souvenir shop."

To obtain enough breast milk for the five infants was a challenge. Marg Neilson remembers it well:

> As part of our training we worked in the hospital's dairy where the protein and lactic acid milks were prepared for babies on special diets. Every night for several months we had to send breast milk to North Bay for the infant Quints. There were a lot of women who had milk to spare — even those nursing their own babies. It was amazing. Tiny little women would proudly bring in big bottles full of milk. They'd bring it in the morning and then we'd sterilize and pack it for the night train.

Pasteurization in Ontario

The second major event was pasteurization. Although Toronto had had pasteurized milk since 1911, many patients at Sick Kids' came from other parts of the province suffering from tuberculosis, the result of drinking infected milk.

Alan Brown never hesitated to seize an opportunity. In the spring of 1935 he was seated beside Mitchell Hepburn, the premier of Ontario, at a formal dinner. Hepburn was just as blunt and decisive as the man sitting at his side. As soon as he had become Premier he had fired many of the civil servants appointed by the former Tory government. "Mitch" survived only one term as Premier. He was not popular with the people of Ontario and he knew it but, like Brown, he did not care.

Brusquely and eloquently Alan Brown described the tragic and unnecessary plight of his out-of-town patients suffering the effects of bovine tuberculosis. Mitch listened closely while Alan damned the situation as a disgrace to the province, a province so fearful of its farmers' wrath that children were forced to suffer the consequences of unpasteurized milk. He slyly added that because there were no farmers in Toronto the city children had been drinking safe milk for twenty-five years. He finished his lecture to the Premier with characteristic showmanship; he challenged Mitch to accompany him through the wards to see for himself the ravages of bovine bone and joint tuberculosis.

Hepburn accepted the challenge and was shocked by the deformed bodies he saw as he walked past the cots. He returned to the Parliament Buildings in Queen's Park and with his usual decisiveness immediately had a bill prepared to enforce pasteurization throughout the province. He was a farmer himself and his riding, Elgin County, a farming community. He knew his farmers would howl in protest; they would not want to be put to the trouble and expense of pasteurization. Nevertheless, like Alan Brown, he did not hesitate to do what was urgently needed even when his reward was an infuriated constituency. Brown and Hepburn were an unlikely team, but together they were responsible for the elimination of bovine tuberculosis from the province. It was the largest geographical area in the world to enforce such a law at that time.

Poliomyelitis

The third major event during the depression years was the 1937 polio epidemic, far worse than that of 1930 and the most severe the province has ever suffered. The resources and staff of The Hospital for Sick Children were pushed almost beyond their capacity. Everyone pitched in to confront the emergency. With a child already in the hospital's only respirator and with cases multiplying daily, Superintendent Joe Bower confidently undertook to construct "iron lungs" using the hospital's respirator as a model. He had already attempted to obtain one or two from hospitals as far away as Boston without success. All were in use. Working round the clock in a makeshift workshop set up in the tunnel that ran from the back to the front of the hospital, Joe, with Harry Balmforth and his team of welders and carpenters, gave up their summer holidays to construct a rough but effective iron lung every twenty-four hours.

Overcrowding became acute; even the hallways were filled with parents waiting to have their children examined. The slightest headache, cold or fever, however innocuous, was feared as the first sign of the disease. They were lined up on Elizabeth Street and along the corridors. It was hectic:

> The resident interns were up all day and all night. I remember Bill Hawke saying, "This is nonsense. The residents have to get some sleep." He organized shifts and the attending medical staff took over and did lumbar punctures for four or five hours in rotation. We did about seven hundred a week and a lot of them were positive, a lot of them.[38]

Laurie Chute had just finished his internship. The government provided him with a car and diagnostic equipment, including a microscope. He drove around the countryside as far as Barrie doing lumbar punctures on children and adults with suspicious symptoms to identify patients with abnormally high white blood counts in the cerebrospinal fluid.

Alan Brown, now fifty years old, pushed himself without mercy. The fear of contagion was so great that schools remained closed till the middle of October when the epidemic began to die out with the first frosts. Until then he prudently kept his family isolated up at his old log cabin on Ahmic Lake along the Magnetawan River, rarely able to spend even a night or two with them.

Alan Brown in Demand
During the twenties and thirties his renown in Canada grew to the point where he was the consultant to everybody involved with children. No decision was made without his advice. He was Director of Child Hygiene for Toronto, consulting physician to the local, provincial and federal departments of health, the Infants' Home (now part of the Childrens' Aid Society), Riverdale Isolation Hospital, Women's College Hospital and Toronto General Hospital. The list is almost endless. "He thrived on his reputation of being the saviour of the infants of Ontario."[39]

Sometimes he must have been unnerved by his responsibilities, by his loneliness in his decisions. He was not always as confident as he appeared and many lives depended on the accuracy of his medical judgement; but there was no one at Sick Kids' with his paediatric background and experience whom he felt he could consult.

He pushed the hospital into the community, organizing and assisting in clinics and health programs in the schools, in public recreational

TABLE OF MEASURES AND CALORIC VALUES
1 level tablespoon = 3 level teaspoons

1 ounce by volume of Corn Syrup = 2 tablespoons =	140 calories
1 ounce by weight of Lactose = 3 level tablespoons =	120 calories
1 ounce by weight of Dextri Maltose = 4 level tablespoons =	120 calories
1 ounce by weight of Dextri Maltose with Vitamin B = 6 level tablespoons =	120 calories
1 ounce by weight of Cane Sugar = 2 level tablespoons =	120 calories
1 ounce by weight of Glucose = 3 level tablespoons =	120 calories
1 ounce by weight of Barley Flour = 4 level tablespoons =	100 calories
1 ounce by weight of Rice Flour = 4 level tablespoons =	100 calories
1 ounce by weight of Casec = 12 level tablespoons =	105 calories
1 ounce by weight of Apple Sauce = 1 rounded tablespoon, unsweetened =	19 calories
1 ounce by weight of Butter = 1 rounded tablespoon =	225 calories
1 ounce by weight of Carrots = 1 rounded tablespoon, cooked =	8 calories
1 ounce by weight of Pablum = 12 level tablespoons =	106 calories
1 ounce by weight of Custard = 1 rounded tablespoon =	29 calories
1 ounce by weight of Meat (scraped) = 1 rounded tablespoon, uncooked =	50 calories
1 ounce by weight of Potato (baked) = 1 rounded tablespoon =	30 calories
1½ ozs. by weight of Spinach = 1 rounded tablespoon, cooked =	4 calories
1 ounce by weight of Bacon = 3 thin slices, cooked crisp =	155 calories
1 ounce by volume = 1 rounded tbsp. expressed, washed, riced Junket Curds =	60 calories
Sunwheat Biscuit =	40 calories
1 ounce of Orange Juice =	12 calories
1 ounce of Tomato Juice =	5 calories
average slice of Bread =	100 calories
Egg =	72 calories
gm. of Fat =	9.3 calories
1 gm. of protein =	4.1 calories
1 gm. of carbohydrate =	4.1 calories

Caloric Requirements Per Pound of Body Weight

1—6 months	50 calories	2 years	35 calories
6—12 months	40 calories	4 years	35 calories
Prematures	65-100 calories	8 years	28 calories
Weaklings and Decomposition	65-100 calories	12 years	23 calories

Form 467—10M—10-8-41

FEEDING CARD
by
ALAN BROWN, M.D.
Physician-in-Chief
Hospital for Sick Children
Professor of Paediatrics
University of Toronto

REQUIREMENTS OF NORMAL INFANTS
Protein Requirement = Protein of 1½ oz. milk per pound body weight daily.
Fat Requirement = Fat of 1½ oz. 4% milk per pound of body weight daily.
Fluid Requirement per 24 hours = 3 oz. per pound up to 40 oz.
Sugar Requirement = 1 oz. under 12 lbs.
Sugar Requirement = 1½ oz. over 12 lbs.

CONCENTRATED FEEDINGS
1 ounce by volume = 1 rounded tbsp. Mead's Cereal (cooked 1 oz. by wt. raw, in 10 ozs. water) = 11 calories.

1 ounce by volume = 1 rounded tbsp. Mead's Cereal (cooked 1 oz. by wt. raw, in 10 ozs. 2% milk) = 26 calories.

Thick Feedings = 1 oz. raw Mead's Cereal to every 10 ozs. liquid formula cooked ½ hour in double boiler.

Dr. Brown's compact, 2-sided "Feeding Card" given to all his mothers

AVERAGE PERCENTAGES AND CALORIC VALUES OF MILK AND MILK PREPARATIONS

WEIGHT				F.	C.	P.	Cal.
BIRTH	Boys	7.6 lbs.	Breast milk	4.0	7.0	1.0	20.0
	Girls	7.2 "	Whole cow's milk	3.5	4.5	3.5	20.0
1st Month	Boys	8.2 "	2% cow's milk	2.0	4.5	3.5	15.0
	Girls	7.7 "	Evaporated milk	7.8	9.9	6.9	43.5
2nd "	Boys	10.7 "	Condensed milk	9.0	53.5	8.1	128.0
	Girls	10.2 "	2% L.A.M. (cultured)	2.0	4.0	3.5	14.0
3rd "	Boys	12.7 "	L.A.M. powd'r	1.8	3.8	3.0	16.0
	Girls	12.2 "	1 oz. (5 level tsp.) to 10 ozs. cold water.				
4th "	Boys	14.2 "	Biolac (for prematures)	4.8	16.4	5.6	38.0
	Girls	13.6 "	1 oz. (8 level tsp.) to 8 ozs. warm water.				
5th "	Boys	15.4 "	Dryco	1.5	5.7	4.0	16.0
	Girls	14.8 "	1 level tsp. to 2 ozs. water.				
6th "	Boys	16.0 "	Hypo-allergic milk	3.3	4.7	3.5	20.0
	Girls	15.5 "	1 oz. (4 level tsp.) to 10 ozs. cold water.				
7th "	Boys	16.7 "	Klim (skimmed)	0.1	5.2	3.7	11.0
	Girls	16.2 "	1 oz. (4 level tsp.) to 10 ozs. cold water.				
8th "	Boys	17.3 "	Klim (whole)	3.3	4.5	3.2	20.0
	Girls	16.8 "	1 oz. (5 level tsp.) to 10 ozs. cold water.				
9th "	Boys	17.7 "	Olac (for prematures)	3.3	7.5	2.7	19.0
	Girls	17.2 "	1 oz. (3½ level tsp.) to 7 ozs. warm water.				
10th "	Boys	18.3 "	Protein milk powder	2.7	2.3	3.7	12.0
	Girls	17.7 "	1 oz. (5 level tsp.) to 11 ozs. cold water.				
11th "	Boys	19.4 "	Similac	3.4	6.8	1.5	19.0
	Girls	18.8 "	1 oz. (4 level tsp.) to 7½ ozs. warm water.				
12th "	Boys	20.5 "	S.M.A.	3.5	7.3	1.3	20.0
	Girls	19.8 "	1 oz. (3½ level tsp.) to 7 ozs. warm water.				
18th "	Boys	22.8 "	S.M.A. protein	2.2	2.8	3.5	15.0
	Girls	22.0 "	1 oz. (4 level tsp.) to 9 ozs. warm water.				
2 Years	Boys	25.4 "	Sobee	2.4	4.8	4.0	16.0
	Girls	25.0 "	1 oz. (6 level tsp.) to 7 ozs. water, and boil.				
3 "	Boys	31.2 "					
	Girls	30.0 "					
4 "	Boys	35.0 "					
	Girls	34.0 "					
5 "	Boys	41.2 "					
	Girls	39.8 "					
6 "	Boys	45.8 "					
	Girls	43.8 "					
7 "	Boys	49.5 "					
	Girls	48.0 "					

1. Cream to be removed with Chapin dipper.
2. Mixtures to be made up to 20, 25, 30, 35 or 40 ounces.
   To obtain 4% milk use whole quart after shaking.
   To obtain 3% milk use remainder after skimming off top 2 ounces.
   To obtain 2% milk use remainder after skimming off top 4 ounces.
   To obtain 1% milk use remainder after skimming off top 8 ounces.
1 ounce of any Sugar by weight in a 20-ounce mixture adds 5% Carbohydrate.
1 ounce of any Starch by weight in a 20-ounce mixture adds 3.5% Carbohydrate.
1 ounce of Corn Syrup by volume in a 20-ounce mixture adds 6.0% Carbohydrate.
½-ounce of Casec by weight in a 20-ounce mixture adds 2% Protein.

NORMAL LABORATORY DETERMINATIONS

Ascorbic acid 7 to 10 mgms. per 100 cc. (optimal).
Calcium 10 to 11 mgms. per 100 cc.
Inorganic phosphorus 5 to 6 mgms. per 100 cc. serum
Chlorides (NaCl) N to 10 to 100.
Cholesterol 150-180 mgms.
Creatinin 1-2 mgms. per 100 cc.
Fat 350 mgms. per 100 cc.
Galactose tolerance - 3 grams
NPN 25-35 mgms. per 100 cc.
Phosphatase 15 units per 100 cc. (King Armstrong)
Serum protein 6-8 grams per 100 cc.
   Oedema level 5 grams per 100 cc.
Sugar 70 to 110 mgms. per 100 cc.
Sugar tolerance not over 160. Fails to normal within 3 hours
Vit. dex. Bench. Under 2 units, or 1 mgm./c.
Prothrombin time - 35 sec. (Quick Method).
Bleed'g time - 5 min. Clotting time - 5 min.
Platelet count 100-300,000.
Sedimentation rate - 10 (micromethod).

			Prophylactic Daily Dose
Thiamin chloride	—333 Int. Units per milligram		6 ozs.
Orange juice	—15 mgms. ascorbic acid per oz.		25-50 mgms
Tomato juice (obtained by sieving canned tomatoes)	—5 mgms. ascorbic acid per oz.		2-4 ozs.
Ascorbic acid			3 teasp.
U.S.P. cod liver oil	— { 600 Int. A units 85 Int. D units } per gram		1-2 teasp.
Mead's cod liver oil	— { 1,500 Int. A units 175 Int. D units } per gram		5 to 10 drops
Viosterol	—10,000 Int. D units per gram		5 to 10 drops
Oleum percomorphum	— { 60,000 Int. A units 8,500 Int. D units } per gram		1 mgm.
Vitamin K	—Intramuscularly		

93

facilities, in fact everywhere children's health and welfare were concerned. His goal was to promote preventive medicine. By persuasion, he started newborn care in all city hospitals and opened twelve Well Baby Clinics manned by HSC personnel who examined the patients free of charge, just as they did in the Sick Kids' clinics and public wards.

The World at War again
The Great Depression was drawing to a close when World War II broke out. Five of the most stressful years of Alan Brown's tenure as Physician-in-Chief at HSC followed its outbreak in September 1939. He was fifty-two years old. For more than ten years John Oille, his cardiologist, had been warning him to slow down. Hitler, Mussolini and Hirohito forced him to ignore his doctor's advice.

Uniforms sprouted everywhere and for the second time in twenty-five years the hospital staff was decimated by the demands of war. Nurses, doctors and general support staff rushed to enlist as France fell and the United Kingdom, unprepared and almost alone, fought against the Axis armies of Hitler's Germany and Mussolini's Italy. Resourceful as ever, Alan Brown recruited teen-age girls to work as volunteer nursing aids. He arranged for nurses to be taught procedures normally carried out by doctors. Vacancies in the resident staff gave Alan Brown the opportunity to appoint more female interns. Three in turn became his chief resident: Juliet Chisholm, 1942-3, Lillian Sugarman Clark, 1943-4 and Jean Davey, 1944-5.

Toronto again became a world of casualty lists. Mail was censored, and gasoline, butter and sugar were rationed. Women worked shifts in munitions factories and the sobriquet "Rosie the riveter" was coined to symbolize their work. Red Cross volunteers prepared parcels for Canadian prisoners of war and Connie Brown's Needlework Guild abandoned baby's bonnets and booties in favour of balaclava helmets and thick wool socks — a rerun of the Guild's contributions in the first war.

Anti-Semitism in the Hospital
Alan Brown has been accused of anti-Semitism. His HSC Jewish staff and other colleagues are emphatic that the accusation is false. In 1940, as Adolph Hitler overran the continent, Brown accepted Dr. Karger, a German citizen and a Jewish paediatrician, fleeing the tyranny of the Nazis. He gave him a job working in Harry Ebbs' basement laboratory

where he would be protected from staff members unsympathetic to him.

After three years' post-graduate training at the Mayo Clinic, a young Jewish doctor returned to Toronto to start a practice in 1935: "I'd made the usual applications but I was in practice for nine years before I was invited to join the staff of Sick Kids'." In those days many of Alan Brown's associates were anti-Semitic. They had not been exposed, as he had been, to the best of Jewish medicine and philanthropy in Berlin, Munich and New York.

The Toronto of those days had the highest proportion of citizens of Anglo-Saxon extraction of any city in North America. Alan Brown was broad-minded in a society so conservative and narrow-minded that the derogatory acronym WASP (white Anglo-Saxon protestant) was later coined to stigmatize its members. Anti-Semitism was common and Alan Brown's lack of prejudice was unusual. Fred Weinberg speaks of Alan Brown's embarrassment at the attitude of the Dean of Medicine, W.E. Gallie. Over the telephone Brown told Gallie he had invited Alton Goldbloom, chief of paediatrics at McGill University and Montreal Children's Hospital, to sit with other honoured guests at the official opening of the new hospital. Weinberg, working beside Brown overheard him reply: "Oh no, Ed! He's not one of those. Yes, he is a Jew and a fine doctor." Goldbloom attended and during the course of the afternoon he mused, "Weinberg, this is unusual — to be a VIP at Sick Kids'."

One HSC staff member is convinced that the anti-Semitism of other members of the staff, especially the prejudice of D.E. Robertson, for many years the chief surgeon of HSC, was the reason Jews had difficulty obtaining staff appointments. Many of his contemporaries remember his declaration: "No Jew will be appointed to this hospital except over my dead body." Evidence of Robertson's attitude can be found in a 1975 article in which Dr. A.I. Willinsky is described as "one of the first and most distinguished Jewish doctors of early Toronto".[40] The article then refers to Willinsky's autobiography in which he described his interview with Dr. D.E. Robertson in 1919 regarding his application to the HSC for an appointment. Robertson is quoted as declaring:

> To be honest with you, they say you would be a good man for the staff here. But you may as well know that I'd hate to see any Jew get in this hospital.[41]

96

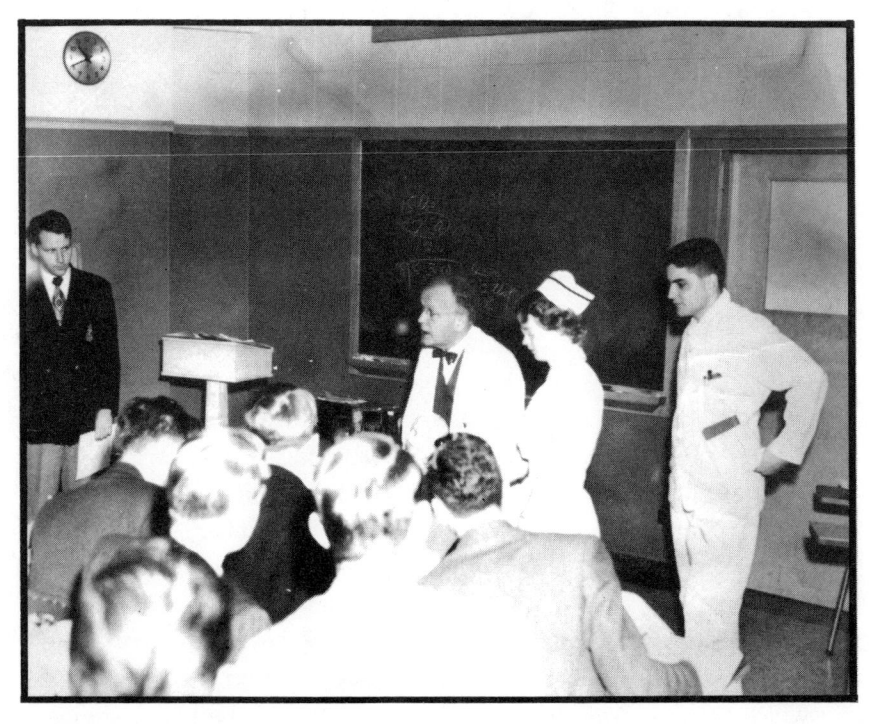

Alan Brown teaching, assisted by nurse, baby and Robert H. Johnson (senior intern in white) in HSC lecture theatre on College Street (photo H.W. Tetlow, courtesy Maclean's Magazine)

Few were as outspoken about their bias as "DE" appears to have been. For whatever reason, Brown refrained from tilting with Robertson over the Jewish issue. With the exception of the appointment of Lillian Clark (née Sugarman) as Alan Brown's Chief Resident in 1943 when the hospital was short-staffed during World War II, a second Jewish appointment was not offered until after Robertson's death in 1944. Since that date the number of HSC interns and staff members of the Jewish faith has increased considerably, and today anti-Semitic discrimination does not exist at Sick Kids'.

> The day after Eddy Robertson died Alan Brown telephoned to ask me for lunch. I KNOW he had no anti-Semitic feelings. He understood and respected the Jewish holidays but he used to tease me about choosing ham for the menu of the staff suppers I had to organize for him.[42]
> — No, he was certainly not anti-Semitic. I cherish the memories of my time with him. He treated me like a lady no matter how upset or angry he was.[43]

Alan Brown's lack of prejudice manifested itself clearly in his attitude towards his Jewish professors, colleagues and acquaintances for whom he had the greatest respect.

Part Six — The Professor and his Students

In 1919, when he was appointed Physician-in-Chief of The Hospital for Sick Children and the University of Toronto's Professor of Paediatrics, Alan Brown was determined to share his extensive training, knowledge and experience with his staff and students. He would teach them everything he could in the few hours allotted to paediatric classes. In those days, until well after World War II, most of his students went out into the world as general practitioners treating both adults and children. He wanted to send them forth equipped to recognize and treat their patients' medical problems but know when to seek help in difficult cases. He often said their reputations would wax or wane with their skill in paediatrics and obstetrics. Margaret Neilson, RN, would hear former students say, "I really didn't know how much I was learning from him till I got out in practice." Inspired by Alan Brown's dedication and enthusiasm, some of his students followed him into paediatrics in order to have the opportunity of further study under him. At one time he had trained sixty to seventy-five percent of the paediatricians in Canada according to his nursing and medical staff interviewed.

Several assistants prepared his classes and clinics. The chief resident or a senior intern, with the head nurse of either the infants' (up to age two) or the children's wards (to age twelve) would choose the patients and arrange to have them brought down to the lecture theatre:

> He liked to show the babies at different ages, different stages of development, what to expect of them, how they should be fed. He would go through the normal characteristics of a child and then would talk about symptoms and how to diagnose and treat any problems. The course went through a logical sequence from normal to abnormal conditions. It was very carefully thought out. Sometimes he would have to change his topic according to the babies available.

He was fond of using realistic wax models he'd brought from Germany to illustrate various rashes and skin diseases. On one occasion a child was whisked off for a non-emergency operation just before Alan Brown was to lecture on the case. He was furious. He roared at the chief surgical resident for not having waited until after his class, forcing him to substitute another topic at the last moment. There were nearly always patients available to illustrate the various conditions brought about by improper or contaminated feeding: coeliac disease, lactose intolerance, gastroenteritis, malnutrition, bovine tuberculosis and many others:

> Dr. Brown liked to put on an act. We had a child who had been brought in to him with "failure to thrive" — a favoured expression in those days. He was about two but the size of a six-month-old baby. I took him into the clinic lying on a stretcher. Dr. Brown asked the students what age they thought this child was; they guessed between six and nine months. After some discussion he gave me the nod. I sat the child up and said to him, "What would you like for lunch?" He replied, "I want meat!" The whole class exploded with laughter. He loved to tease them in this way when he had a chance.[44]

Children's attitudes towards attendance at Alan Brown's lectures is described by Helen McCallum, RN.

> Some of the older children were proud to be chosen for his class but most were scared to death to be brought into the lecture theatre. We tried to calm them by explaining carefully what would happen and why they were there. They were children with heart defects, rheumatic fever, pneumonia, rickets and all sorts of conditions we don't see anymore.

Student reactions to Alan Brown's teaching:

> — He didn't waste time. You felt what he was telling you came straight from God.
> — He had a fetish for the spectacular.
> — One aspect of his teaching was cruel. Sure, it made an impression on you but it wasn't nice. He'd take a student and lead him on to the wrong conclusion and then make a sarcastic remark about how stupid he was. This method made you remember but it wouldn't go down well today and it didn't with our class then. One day he brought in a pretty little baby and after several students examined it, he asked each one in turn, "Would you adopt it? Would you?" Forced to reply they hesitated, "Well, yes, maybe." Then he roared, "You fools, this is a mongoloid. Better to leave it in the infectious ward!" Such remarks are hardly in keeping with the caring aspect of medicine.
> — He really was a tormentor of students, his scathing remarks insulting.
> — He had his students terrified. He loved to get them in a corner and embarrass them.

Thoughts would scatter under his attacks. Few had the courage to stand up to him. Those who did would earn his respect if they could prove their point.

> — He was a superb lecturer. His classes were lively. You certainly didn't fall asleep and he really put paediatrics on the map here; there's no doubt about that. But he was a very

unpleasant character. I think a lot of his staff hated him and when I joined his fraternity I got the impression he was not popular.
— As a student and intern I found him crotchety, strict, but a fine teacher. If he asked you a question you had to have an immediate answer even if you faked it. But if he caught you, you'd had it.
— He was very demanding. As chief resident I had to oversee the final-year students, assign cases to them and make sure they were ready to present them. I remember how cruel and savage he could be. Behind that I saw a soft, gentle type of person.
— He really was two different people — not exactly Jekyll and Hyde, but when you got Alan away from the profession he was delightful, pleasant, friendly. At the hospital it was a different story.

A young doctor applied for an appointment to the HSC staff:

I walked along with him towards the infants' ward where some of his staff and residents were waiting and politely said, "I apologize for delaying you; your doctors are waiting for you." He snapped, "Let them wait."

One of his residents who liked and respected him had to admit that he was rude, sarcastic, strict and intolerant with his residents.

Margaret Neilson describes his effect on students:

He really took advantage of those he thought were frightened of him. If he saw they were terribly nervous or trying to escape, he would pick on them. Some were so flustered they weren't able to take in what he was saying. I used to give the boys a few tips: "When you get up to present your case, put your notes on the lectern, don't hold them in your hand so he can see it shaking."

A vigorous description comes from Dr. Morton Shulman, who is not easily browbeaten:

He had a terrible temper, a reputation bigger than God's and I didn't learn a thing from him. I was too terrified. He'd pick on a student and completely demolish him.

There were mixed reactions to Alan Brown's teaching:

- He bullied those who didn't have the answers. He was always threatening to flunk you. But there's nothing like a little fear to keep you on your toes.
- When I was a student he intimidated and ridiculed me. That was his method.
- He didn't believe in psychiatry. In a public lecture he told the story of a little boy who had a bit of manure he was rolling around in his hands. His mother saw him and said, "Johnny, what on earth are you doing with that stuff?" "Oh, it's OK, Mum, I'm just making a psychiatrist."

Some comments on his teaching techniques were favourable:

- He trained students and junior staff very well but he had a tremendous ego. . . .
- I'd like to emphasize that you could argue with him; you could get your ideas across to him. Even as a student, if you stood your ground and could put forth arguments for your case, he would listen to you — he listened very well. I have nothing but very fond memories of Dr. Brown, even as a student. For example, we'd have to present a case to the class. To make the right diagnosis, we'd examine the patient but we'd also need the history. You couldn't question the patients because they were too young. You'd have to get the history from the patient's chart. Now Alan was very cute. He would take a big black grease pencil and he'd strike out the diagnosis and all the comments he'd written on the chart. The history itself was there as taken from the parents but you couldn't read anything else. The student had to start from scratch. Some of them would get alcohol or ether and wipe the black grease paint off the chart. But if they showed too much knowledge of what was underneath the paint he'd catch them up

as he grilled them or he'd throw in something else that hadn't been put on the chart and trap them that way. It was almost impossible to fool Alan; he was too sharp.
— I don't think any intern comes out now with the clinical acumen that he taught us — nobody. We see the Sick Kids' students all the time so we know.

The admiration and respect that his teaching commanded waned towards the end of his career:

— He was a dogmatic teacher and did not indulge in much that was truly scientific.
— I don't know what to say about his teaching. We had respect for him and what he had accomplished. That alone made us sit up and listen. But he wasn't as good as I thought he would be. He was dogmatic and inflexible. Medicine was changing rapidly at that time (1949) and we wondered, was he really with it? Was he really up to date? As students it was difficult for us to judge.

By the time the Class of '50 came along Alan Brown had given so much of himself for so long that he had little left to give. He was sixty-three years old and his health was failing. His colleague and friend Nelles Silverthorne, reflects, "Sometimes he was away and when he returned he'd say to me, 'Just a little atherosclerosis'."

Part 7 — Conferences, Publications, Plagiarism

During the twenties and thirties, Alan Brown became a household name in Canada. His huge private practice and the long hours he worked in the hospital left him little time or energy to write papers or attend medical conferences. He is given credit as the sole author of only one book. He published few original research studies. He was not as well known internationally as the hospital he promoted or some of the medical staff he hired, such as Fred Tisdall, Theo Drake, Harry Ebbs and Nelles Silverthorne. Several of his staff members admit that Alan Brown has not received the lasting recognition they thought he would.

He rarely went to medical conferences and attended only when he thought he might receive information of relevance to his hospital work and his practice:

> Though not really shy, Alan was uncomfortable in large gatherings, social or professional. He got the latest in medical developments from the journals he read constantly. Fred (Tisdall) was just the opposite. He was a "joiner" and a sociable man and had close contacts in the business community. He thought medical conferences were important, as much for the contacts he made as for the latest in medical discoveries.[45]

Publications and Plagiarism

As the Physician-in-Chief of The Hospital for Sick Children he expected to be listed as a co-author of all the books and papers written in the Department of Medicine during his tenure. A bibliography of the publications Alan Brown "co-authored" over nearly thirty-two years as Chief of Medicine would be misleading. The list would contain several hundred titles unjustifiably attributed to him. Some doubted he even read the papers before publication and were annoyed that his name was listed as author when he had little or nothing to do with the publication. Others treated the matter with resignation or excused him because they respected him as the father of paediatrics in Canada. The practice of including the name of the departmental head on all papers coming out of a department was a carry-over from the British and German tradition. It was almost universal and lingered until after World War II. Even today, in quite reputable centres, it is not uncommon for names to appear in the list of authors merely as a courtesy for their consent to the inclusion of their patients in a study. The names of eminent physicians in Canada, the United States and Europe appear on so many publications that they couldn't possibly have done more than pat the heads of the brilliant juniors who wrote them.

Many of Alan Brown's staff acknowledge that he was permanently blackballed by the prestigious American Pediatric Society because of plagiarism in a paper that bore his name. One of his colleagues suggests the Society's boycott may have been due to its disapproval of Alan Brown's insistence on his co-authorship of *all* the papers published by the HSC staff rather than the plagiarization of one. A young paediatrician at Sick Kids' applying to hospitals in New York for a residency in 1933, was shocked to find a lack of respect for Alan Brown:

I first went to the Babies' Hospital where Dr. Ashley Weech asked who had written on my behalf. I showed him my three letters. He read them and handed them back saying, "I would suggest that you keep this one in your pocket when you go to have your interviews." It was the letter from Dr. Brown. Dr. Weech then told me that Alan had put himself in disfavour with the paediatric fraternity in the United States when he took Miss Angelia Courtney to Toronto where some of the papers he wrote with her there contained research which she had done prior to going to Toronto in 1921. As a result of this, he was permanently blackballed from membership in the American Pediatric Society.[46]

Jack Slavens, an HSC staff member of twenty-five years standing, has a different explanation:

Alan had written a paper on the bacterial count of stools.[47] He had plagiarized the material and published it under his own name. He was intellectually dishonest, morally dishonest. So he was blackballed. He was a good clinician but not a good scientist. In his published papers he rode on the coattails of others and as the Professor of Paediatrics and head of the Hospital he could get away with it.

In the first three editions of *The Normal Child* (1923, 1926 and 1932), Brown's name appears as the sole author. In the preface he does not name his staff members who wrote whole sections. He states: "This volume is presented . . . with no claim for original material beyond that obtained from an extensive hospital and private practice." In the 1948 and 1958 editions the contributions of Dr. Elizabeth Chant Robertson are acknowledged. Her name shares the title page with his as co-author.

On the spine and the title page of *Common Procedures in the Practice of Paediatrics* (1926, 1932, 1939 editions), Brown and Tisdall, in that order, are shown as the authors. On a 1943 Toronto Academy of Medicine data form filled in by its Fellows, Brown describes himself as "Senior Author with F.F. Tisdall" of *Common Procedures*. Mary Tisdall confesses that Fred wrote it but she allows that Alan, as Physician-in-Chief of the hospital, was appropriately listed as first author. Tisdall's son Charles disagrees: "Alan Brown had nothing to do with it. My father wrote that book. But

Brown was a determined old bugger. He even tried to interfere with our arrangements for Dad's funeral!" In the preface to *Common Procedures* Brown and Tisdall "express their indebtedness" to several staff doctors, among them a bitter T.G.H. Drake who had understood he was to be cited as third author. "Theo was really annoyed about that. He said he was a young man then and needed the credit."[48] Fred Tisdall tried to make amends by writing on the flyleaf of the copy he presented to Drake: *To Dr. T.G.H. Drake, at whose suggestion this book was written, who wrote Chapters six and ten in their entirety and who greatly assisted in the compilation of the other chapters. . . January 15, 1927.*[49]

Alan Brown's habit of taking credit for the work of others was so notorious that sometimes his staff made fun of it. At the annual meeting of the Canadian Medical Association in 1940 he gave the fourth Blackader Lecture, "A Decade of Paediatric Progress". He did not acknowledge his indebtedness to the eleven staff members who had written the various sections for him.[50] He gave it as his own. Before the meeting they joked that they ought to go and sit in the front row and when he came to their sections they would get up in turn, bow and sit down again.

— Chapter 6 —

Private Practice

The Cycling Whippersnapper

As soon as he returned to Toronto in June of 1914, Alan Brown opened an office in his home, a lower duplex at 440 Avenue Road on the corner of Balmoral Avenue. His practice grew slowly but steadily. The recommendations of associates who had been students with him attracted parents to him. Many patients were brought by mothers who had heard of "the new baby doctor in town" through his wife's extensive family and their connections to "old Toronto". He amused some of the social set by making house calls on the rusty old bicycle he had ridden in his undergraduate days.

The Smith family lived in a lovely old farmhouse in the middle of the city. Fruit trees dotted its spacious lawns on the north side of Glen Elm Avenue. They first encountered Alan Brown when he was on call for their family doctor, H.T. Machell. Their daughter, Gin, was one year old, sickly and weighed only twelve pounds. When Alan arrived on his bicycle to examine the baby, Mrs. Smith took one look at him and burst into tears. She had no faith in the medical ability of one so young and was certain her child would die. Ignoring her distress Alan Brown immediately took control of the situation. Watchful and wary, but finally impressed by his self-confidence and blunt approach, Mrs. Smith was reassured. She obeyed his detailed feeding instructions, spending hours in the kitchen preparing various chopped, mushy dishes. With the new diet Gin began to gain weight, and when Dr. Machell returned from his holidays the Smiths informed him that henceforth, they would take their children to Dr. Alan Brown.[1] Dr. Machell's reaction is not recorded but he was close to retirement. Brown knew it was a breach of professional etiquette to "steal" a patient from a colleague for whom he'd been on call, but the Smiths had been insistent. Gin was their child and it was their right, they said, to change doctors. Perversely, Brown was less inclined to accept a parent's right to remove a baby from *his* care to a rival.

Stories of the shift from the general practice family doctors to the new baby doctor were legion and did not increase his popularity with the abandoned physicians. He didn't care; the health of children was his first consideration. Stories of his idiosyncrasies only raised his profile and attracted patients to his practice. He had too many house calls to take time to knock or ring door bells. He just swept in and went straight upstairs to his patient. Sometimes he found himself in the wrong house but, unfazed, he just rushed out again. Once he burst into the bedroom of a naked woman who was definitely not his patient. The sheepish doctor made one of his rare apologies as he beat a hasty retreat.

His first office was in the dining room. One of his nieces, Elisabeth Fisher Lawson, remembers those days when the Browns returned from Germany:

> I stayed with them while my mother had her babies. I was six years old the first time. Uncle Alan had his office in their Balmoral duplex and Auntie Conn had to give up her living and dining rooms to the patients in the afternoons.

Connie Brown handled their finances and, while the practice was growing, used some of her independent income to supplement the patients' fees. Until they could afford an old typewriter, she wrote out his instructions for the patients in long hand. Havergal College had failed to teach Connie to write legibly, causing much bewilderment among parents who had tried to read her handwriting.

Arrival of Grace Haldenby

Alan Brown's rising renown in the hospital, in the community and among grateful parents resulted in the development of a large private practice out of which he was able to subsidize the long hours he worked as a

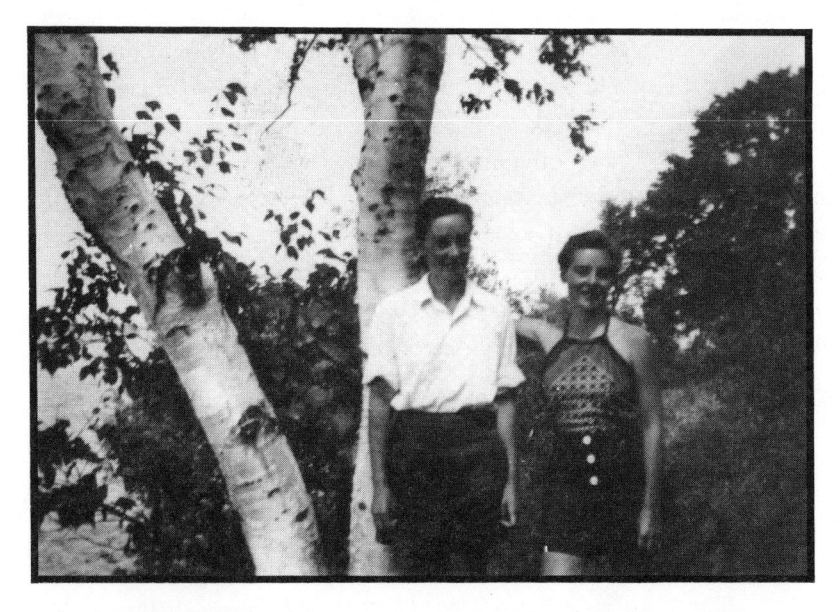

Grace Haldenby (left) with her sister Ruth Mulholland, 1938

"volunteer" in the hospital. Soon a second secretary was needed to assist Miss Tessie Rickard. On her twenty-first birthday in 1927, Miss Grace Haldenby began her long and close association with Alan Brown. He never had any idea what made her tick nor did he take any interest in her personal life. In their thirty-one years together, neither ever acknowledged the other's birthday nor exchanged gifts or cards at Christmas.[2]

There were three Haldenby sisters, two of whom worked for Alan Brown. Doris, who died in 1982, knew the Browns quite well. As a nurse she stayed in the Dunvegan Road house while attending a family member. In the mid-thirties it was Alan himself she looked after while he was recovering from pneumonia contracted on his train trip home after a visit to the Dionne quintuplets. In the mid-Forties Doris retired from the Sick Kids' to work with her sister Grace in Alan Brown's office in the Medical Arts Building. The third sister, Ruth Mulholland spared nothing in her praise for her sisters, especially Grace. She related how Grace's quiet efficiency and warmth drew an affectionate response from mothers and patients waiting their turn to see the doctor. Ruth thought Alan Brown overworked and underpaid her sisters and did not fully appreciate that they were responsible for a smooth-running office. Ruth described her sisters' contributions to Alan Brown's busy private practice in a way that Grace was too modest even to recognize. Mothers depended and responded to her quiet sympathy and help as she and her sister strove to attend to the demands of both doctor and children during their office visits.

Now a delightful old woman in her eighties, Grace reminisced over some of the ups and downs in her working life with Alan Brown. Her love for the children and the respect she had for Brown *as a doctor* persuaded her to remain with him year after year until the final day when she and Doris closed his Medical Arts office forever.

> I was happy with my work — I think. That's why I stayed, though I didn't always approve of what he did and I don't think I ever really liked him.

In all their years together Grace remembered only one time when they tossed aside their professional roles and laughed together as friends. One morning when he arrived she and Doris noticed that

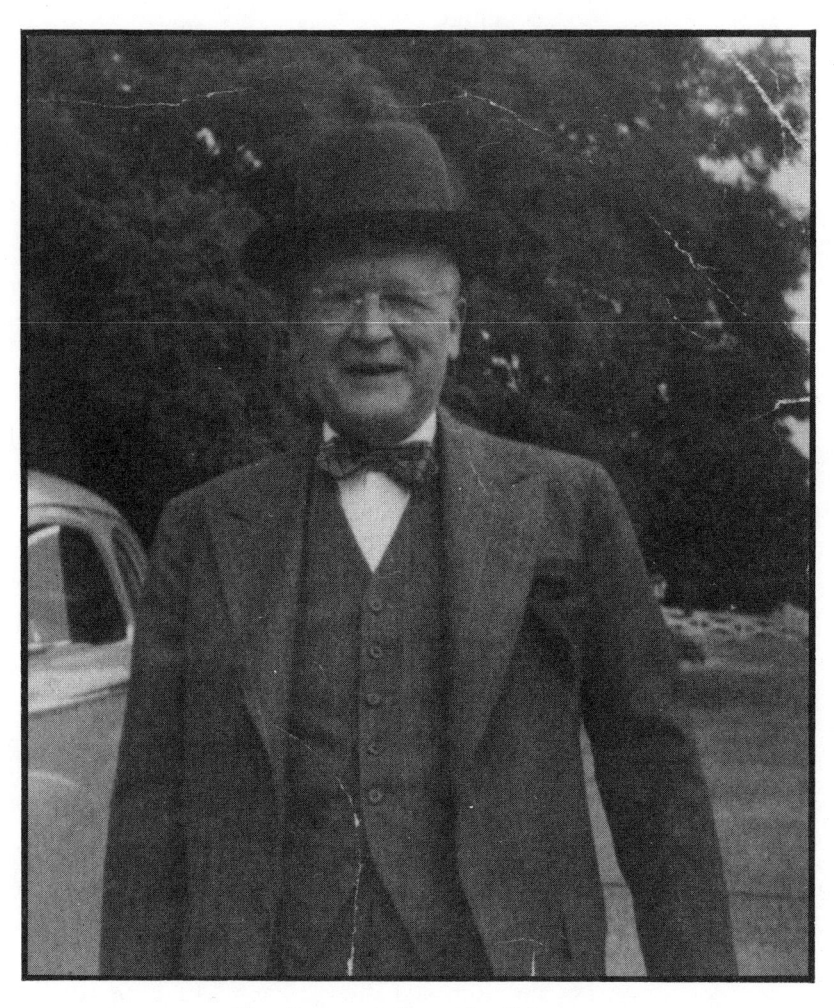

Alan Brown at the peak of his power

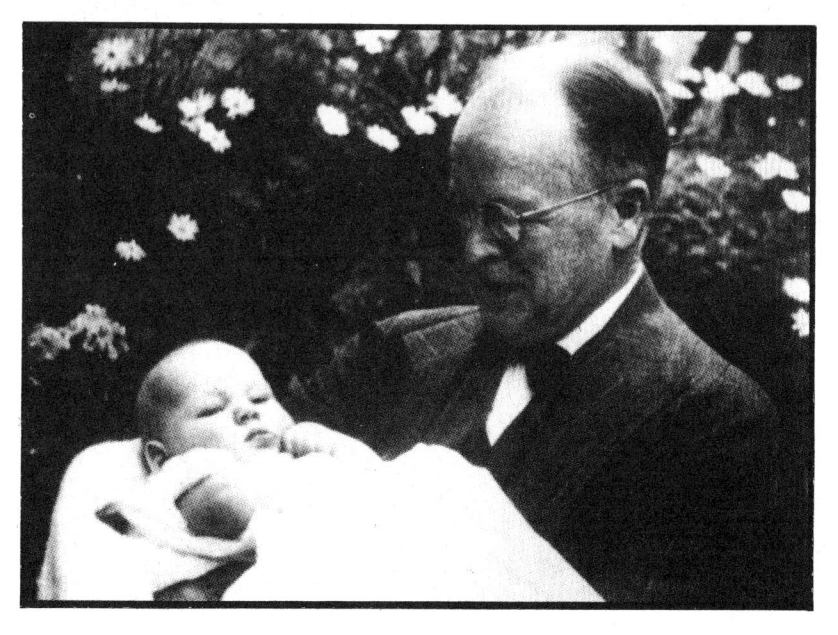

Dr. Alan Brown with Eddy Baker's daughter, Nancy. (Courtesy Hospital for Sick Children)

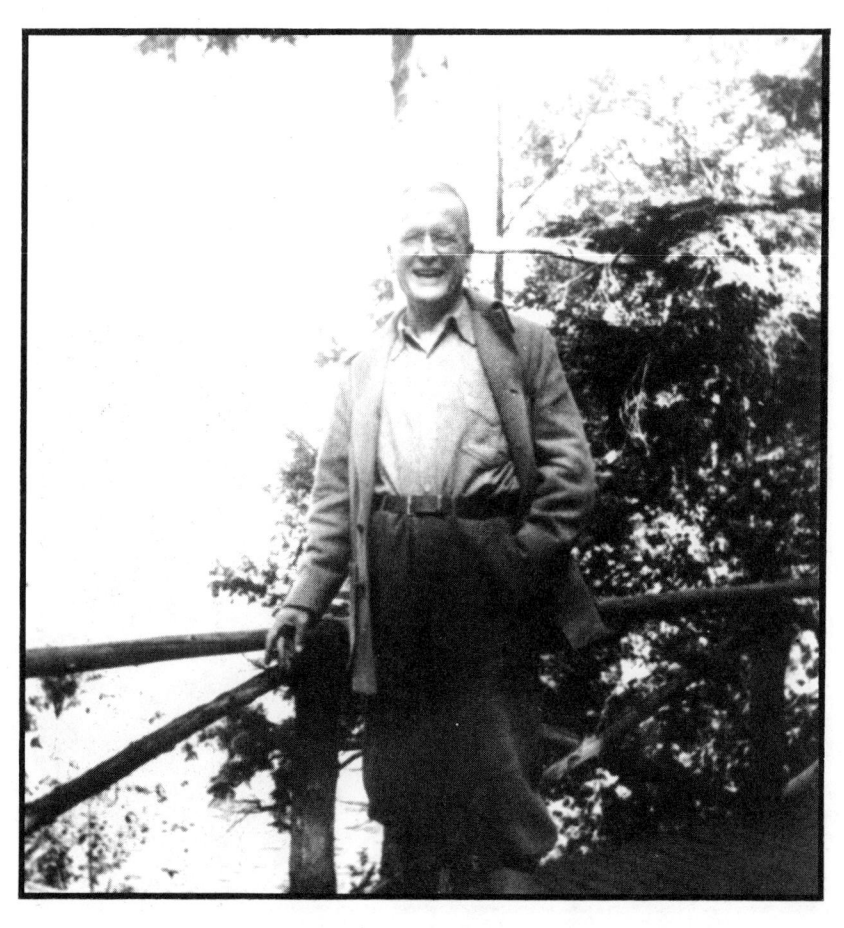

Alan at his cabin overlooking Lake Ahmic, 1942

there was something rather odd about his pants. I think the seam had gone or he'd done his fly up wrong, or something. Anyway, they looked funny. I nudged Doris, "Look, he's coming out." We started to laugh. He turned around and Doris told him there was a hole in his pants. Chuckling and joining in the fun he looked down, then up, and sheepishly asked, "Can you see ME?" His sense of humour was unexpected but did surface once in a while.

At the end of each day after he had rushed off to make his house calls, Doris and Grace would relax for a bit to poke fun at the way their pompous little doctor had boosted his ego that day. Laughing at him broke the tension of their long hours.

He was not really rude but awfully abrupt. He'd come in the door and order, "Get D.E. on the line," as he hung up his hat and coat. And he'd fly off the handle at anything unexpected. He had a quick temper and he knew it. And he was very pigheaded.

Excerpts from Grace's diary:

Jan. 6, 1938 — Dr. B. thoroughly objectionable.
Jan. 14, 1938 — Dr. B. pretty objectionable all week.

Ten years later the diary again indicates exasperation:

May 20, 1949 — busy at the office — told Dr. B. I was going home — it was more than I could take.

Ruth's notation in the diary beside this entry states: "Doris could be difficult — they were both driving Grace crazy." This became apparent in another entry written when Grace was advised by her doctor to resign:

Feb. 20, 1951 — Dr. Hurst Brown took my blood pressure — said I should leave — that did get Alan a bit stirred up. This man (Dr. Hurst Brown) was pretty cute. He knew the situation and he knew Alan Brown. He was pulling a fast one, I don't mind telling you.

For some time after that the atmosphere in the office was uncharacteristically peaceful. Grace's duties remained the same, but Brown didn't demand the impossible. A few weeks later when Grace underwent minor surgery at the Toronto General, Alan Brown even crossed the road to visit her. But it wasn't long before the days slipped back into their usual hectic state:

June 12, 1953 — worked late, till nine or after, every night this week.

Almost two years after his retirement as Chief Physician of HSC his private practice was as busy as ever.

Grace Haldenby's career began in 1927 at the office at 217 St. Clair Avenue West. It didn't have a proper waiting room. The patients sat or stood in the hall where there was a window seat and some little painted wooden chairs with coloured nursery rhyme drawings on the backs. There was a small wooden music box on a table and on the mantelpiece sat a clock. The time it told was seldom correct and its chiming was always off. The clock had been a wedding present and its ever-increasing eccentricities had outlived Mrs. Brown's patience. Alan obediently took it, as ordered, to the office. It disappeared during the later (1932) move to the Medical Arts Building where there was no mantelpiece.

Shortly after the move, a grateful patient gave Alan Brown a child's musical chair. It relieved the children's boredom and deflected their urge towards destruction. Grace reminisces:

— It was Swiss, a lovely little thing made of wood stained dark brown with a standing bear carved in the middle of the back. When a child sat down the chair played Brahm's lullaby — I can almost hear it now: "Lullaby, and good night . . . ." It didn't put the children to sleep but it did take the starch out of them for a bit.

— The waiting room was always in a constant uproar (Ruth remembers). I'd look up to see a child with animal feet racing around the room, his mother's stiff leather gloves pulled over his socks. Other kids would pile the little chairs into rickety towers.

— If you don't believe in hell, you've never been in a paediatric office when it was full of restless kids whooping or weeping or sticking pins in the electric sockets.[3]

Behaviour with Children
Once inside Dr. Brown's inner office the story was different. There was fun in his voice for he delighted children when he spoke their language. Shrieks of laughter could often be heard coming from the examining room. He didn't always let them see his affection for them. His determination to keep them in good health and give them a strong start in life often caused him to conceal his true feelings behind an impatient and gruff manner.

Two little boys at Upper Canada College were asked by their teacher to try to describe God's appearance. One of them replied, "Like Dr. Alan Brown." When their mother related the story to Dr. Brown he laughed so hard he had to wipe his eyes and blow his nose. It put him in excellent humour for the rest of the day and he regaled his family with the story at dinner that night.

But some children were simply terrified when he poked and prodded them in the examining room. He was abrupt and he could hurt, and he could frighten them in his preoccupation for their welfare. With a child who had a lingering illness he was patient and gentle. One boy of eight (now in his mid-seventies) remembers Dr. Brown with affection although his three brothers do not:

> I always felt comfortable with him. He was definite, he was kind and he was funny. Mother said he saved my life so maybe that's why he treated me differently.

Attitude towards Parents
Brown had no patience with mothers who disobeyed his orders. He bullied and insulted them and often reduced them to tears. His intolerance of carelessness, neglect, ignorance or stupidity knew no limits. When a woman rang him at home to ask what she should do for her child's cold his temper flared. "Blow his nose," he ordered, and banged down the receiver. To another who objected to her child undergoing a tonsillectomy in winter, he replied, "We do it indoors now, you know." Parents were unaware of the scathing remarks he wrote on their children's charts when he was fed up with their mothers. "This woman is an idiot." Or

"Tell this featherbrain something? Forget it. It goes in one ear and out both." Or "What a knucklehead. Solid bone, no brain." Or "Mrs. X is a hopeless halfwit." Not surprisingly, many mothers hated him, but their husbands made them keep the appointments.[4]

The majority of parents, however, had complete faith in him in spite of their fear of his scorn. They religiously followed his "paint-by-number" instructions for cleanliness, diet and treatment, all typed on the sheet that they received at the end of each visit. He established a style of practice which has not become outdated. At home it was the mothers who became the bullies as they followed his directions against opposition from their children. The prescribed iron tonic was detested by many of his patients and often had to be forced down throats by pinching the child's nose almost to the point of suffocation.

In February 1932, Muriel Sparrow arrived for a scheduled six-month check-up with her six-year-old daughter and two-year-old son, Robert, his long hair a mass of thick blond curls. Alan Brown took one look at him and exploded. He was furious. He ordered his secretary to type "Baby Ruth" on Robert's feeding schedule, then sent the mother home in tears. Immediately afterwards she had arranged to have Bobby's photograph taken for *The Toronto Daily Star* where it appeared [5] with two other studies representing the current crop of Toronto's beautiful babies. Before Bobby's next appointment his hair had been cut, and his mother left Alan Brown's office clutching the new "FEEDING SCHEDULE for Baby Robert".

Mutiny of the Mothers

Other mothers, tiring of his tyranny, took their children elsewhere. One was Lady Eaton whose daughters had been patients of Alan Brown's for several years. When he advised an appendectomy for one of them, Lady Eaton was unwittingly caught up in a feud between Brown and Herbert Bruce, the head of surgery at the Wellesley Hospital. Bruce was just as arrogant and impatient as Brown. Both were watchful for any infringement on their territory. Their natural temperaments guaranteed a rocky relationship, watched with much amusement by the medical and surgical fraternities as the sparks flared between them.

When Lady Eaton asked Dr. Bruce to perform the operation in the Wellesley the fat was in the fire. Alan Brown wanted D.E. Robertson to operate at Sick Kids'. There is no doubt Dr. Robertson had more experience with this operation — the HSC chief would order appendectomies for almost any child "who failed to thrive". Dr. Bruce ridiculed the frequency of these appendectomies citing them as "Alan Brown's chronic remunerative appendices". The term was bandied about by the medical fraternity in great glee: "Well, old Herbie has won this round," was the consensus as, at Lady Eaton's insistence, the operation was performed by Dr. Bruce at the Wellesley.

To avoid further friction with Alan Brown she regretfully decided to switch Florence Mary and Evelyn to his disciple, Nelles Silverthorne. Silverthorne was thrown into consternation by the request coming directly from Lady Eaton instead of through Brown, and without his knowledge. At that time Brown gave his office over to Silverthorne in the mornings. "He was very generous. He wouldn't let me pay him a cent." As luck would have it, the Eatons were just leaving the office as Alan Brown arrived to see his afternoon patients. Puzzled, he queried Silverthorne, "What are they doing here?" "She asked me if I'd see the girls and I felt I couldn't say no." "Well, If she wants to go to you, she can." He was almost gracious and Silverthorne was stunned. He was expecting one of Alan Brown's famous explosions.

Over the years, there were other mothers who broke ranks. They refused to be bullied and treated discourteously. On one occasion, when Alan Brown was in a bad mood and more insensitive than usual, he tried to intimidate a feisty war bride. He had met his match. The granddaughter of David Lloyd George is not easily intimidated:

Bob was in the Navy and we were stationed in Victoria. I was pregnant and very pleased with myself. When Bob was transferred to Halifax I returned to Toronto, instructed to get Dr. Alan Brown as our paediatrician. Bob then left to join his ship and a couple of weeks later I went into labour. I was twenty-one years old and all alone. My family were in Wales and Bob was at sea somewhere in the Mediterranean and couldn't be reached by cable. I was two days in labour. It was difficult. But after the baby finally arrived I was on top of the world and resting in my hospital bed when the door opened and a small man poked his head in. He just stood there, looked at me and barked, "Cow's milk is for calves." Startled, I said, "I beg your pardon." Then he rudely demanded, "You nurse your baby?" I blew up. "Don't you dare speak to me like that. I have every intention of nursing my baby. I'm a doctor's daughter and a doctor's wife and I was in medicine myself and I know the benefits of nursing a baby. Besides, who the hell are you?" "I'm Dr. Alan Brown." "Oh, you're the paediatrician. Well, is my baby healthy?" He didn't answer me. He just repeated, "Cow's milk is for calves," and closed the door. I thought he was the rudest and cruellest man I'd ever met.[6]

In spite of this awkward beginning to their relationship, the Mac-Millans continued to take their children to Alan Brown until

we had one more episode that finished us. My mother was here from Wales to help with Tommy's birth. She offered to take Anne to Dr. Brown for a checkup. In his office she reported, "I think she's better, she's eating and putting on weight." Now my mother is a rather large woman. Alan Brown turned and looked at her. "Yes," he said. "She's getting almost as fat as her grandmother." Outraged, Mother shot back, "I've travelled all over the world and lived in many countries and I've never in my life met a man as rude as you. Good afternoon." She picked Anne up and walked out. I think he felt a bit badly because his wife 'phoned a few days later to ask mother to play bridge. (Lady Olwen declined.) After that we'd had enough of Dr. Alan Brown. Bob looked after the children.

To offset those who deserted him, there were hundreds of mothers who were happy to know that their children were in the hands of the best paediatrician in Toronto. This alone convinced them to submit to his tyranny. Besides, he was not always fierce with them. On one occasion, Dr. Brown was advising a young woman worried about her daughter's thumb sucking. He asked her to hold her own thumb up in the air and then said, "Stick it in your mouth and give it a good suck." She did so. Dr. Brown looked at her with a twinkle in his eye, "Tastes pretty good doesn't it?" On the other hand he had the habit of frightening young mothers. He'd pick up a baby by the feet and if the mother made a dive for it he'd consider her the nervous type to be treated accordingly.

In the flapper era of The Roaring Twenties, flat chests were *de rigueur* and those whom nature had over-endowed suffered in the name of fashion by binding their bosoms to the point of discomfort. On one occasion Alan Brown abandoned a socialite mother who refused to nurse her baby. He warned her that none of his staff would look after her. Returning to the Sick Kids' he announced, "Mrs. So-and-so has a new baby over at the General. She refuses to breast feed. I do not expect any of you to look after her." At that time if new-born babies weren't breast-fed their chances of dying were high. His anger was not inappropriate but the order to his staff was outrageous.

With mothers whom he knew well and whose judgement he trusted, Alan Brown had no need to hide behind such a harsh persona. He treated them as partners in his concern for their children's well-being. This was the human side of the man that the public didn't often see. In 1940, in the Toronto General, a girl was born to one of his former residents, the same Dr. Helen Reid whose persistent campaign four years earlier had exasperated Alan Brown until he had finally admitted defeat and accepted her as an intern. In company with one or two staff men, Alan Brown walked over to visit her. "Let's see what a physiologist and a paediatrician can do," he said to her by way of an introductory pleasantry. Unfortunately, Helen Reid suffered complications and had to remain in hospital for nearly two months. Her husband, Laurie Chute, was overseas and her family out west. Brown often dropped in to see her. When she returned to Saskatchewan to recuperate, he exacted a promise that she would write him once a month to report on the baby. If she let it slide, she would get a letter from him: "Why haven't you written? Is everything all right?"

Three years later Helen Reid returned to Toronto to take a refresher course before returning to her practice. She left her little daughter with her parents. The child developed septic tracheitis. There were no antibiotics other than the sulphonamides at that time and she became dangerously ill. Helen couldn't get a flight west for three days. They were booked solid. But her father was a doctor and Alan phoned him two or three times each day asking if this or that had been done, sometimes suggesting alternatives.

Many recorded incidents show how much he cared about the children. Katy was four years old in the mid-twenties, a decade before the general use of vaccines. She developed whooping cough and then pneumonia. Alan Brown came to the house each day and the nurse employed by her parents carefully followed his instructions. There was no improvement. Her fever continued to rise. She became delirious. By midnight her parents were at their wits' end. They rang Dr. Brown. He came around at once. He and the nurse sat by the little girl's bed applying ice packs and watching her closely throughout the long night. At dawn the fever broke. He came downstairs exhausted and for a brief moment sat on the bottom step with his head in his hands. The anxious parents waited. Finally he looked up at them; "Your child will recover, but I don't know if I've done you a favour." He did not tell them then that he was concerned about possible brain damage from the high fever. His fear was justified, but the support the family gave Katy and each other allowed her to achieve a kind of normal life.

Largely due to his paediatric skill, Alan Brown saved hundreds of infant lives and many of his patients bragged that they had been "Alan Brown babies". Just after World War II Brown had arranged an HSC staff appointment for Dr. S. Sass-Kortsak, a Polish paediatrician and refugee from the Communist regime. When he and his wife arrived in Toronto, the term "Alan Brown babies" at first bewildered Mrs. Sass-Kortsak, but when she discovered the meaning of the phrase she was enchanted by the image of a long parade of hundreds of Alan Brown's babies.

The waiting room was filled by half past twelve. Appointments began at one o'clock and continued until well after four, depending on how many "extras" had to be inserted at the last moment. Then he would see his patients in various hospitals, and later make anywhere from fifteen to twenty-five house calls before going home, often arriving to find his dinner dried up in the oven, his children asleep and his wife at a concert.

William, his first chauffeur, drove him for many years. William's affair with the Browns' parlour maid caused some consternation, but they escaped dismissal by choosing marriage. Many house calls were as far away as London or Port Hope in the days when the highways were often dirt roads. In 1927 when he was called to see a very sick child in Sault Ste. Marie, he did not have time to drive and jumped on a train instead. At least twice William drove him to Detroit to examine one of the Dodge children in whom Alan Brown had diagnosed coeliac disease. In gratitude the family gave him a Chrysler with a folding mattress in the back so that on long trips he and William could take turns sleeping. Once, late at night, when they were racing to see a very sick child in Belleville they were stopped by the police for speeding. Hearing the explanation, the officer waved them on their way. Later, rushing home as dawn was breaking, the same policeman stopped them: "On your way to see another patient I suppose?"

Alan Brown's readiness to go anywhere at any time to see a sick child had a salutary influence on his colleagues in practice. Late one night a patient telephoned their family doctor to report that his child was very ill. The distraught father wanted him to come at once. The family lived "way out in High Park". The doctor asked a few questions, tried to allay the family's fears and said he'd be out early in the morning. Unhappy with this response, the father cried, "Never mind, I'll call Dr. Brown." As Dr. Silverthorne, recounting the story, said; "Alf certainly didn't want THAT so he quickly replied, "I'll be right out."

Alan Brown had no difficulty keeping two, often three assistants busy (and harried) in his private practice; as well as his secretary, Mary Cassidy, in the hospital office where he arrived at seven o'clock every morning. Before he left the hospital for his afternoon office he would give her more assignments than she could easily handle that day. He would then walk or be driven home for a quick lunch of a soft-boiled egg, melba toast and a glass of skim milk. The afternoons and evenings were as full and even more hectic than his mornings at the hospital. There was little respite.

Casual bookkeeping

Bookkeeping practices in the private office were haphazard. Many patients chose to pay in cash. "It was very popular and sometimes he'd take home the dollar bills. The charge for office visits was two dollars; for house calls, three. Often Mrs. Brown would rush in, "Where's the kale? Where's the kale?"* She would scoop up the money, talking all the time and hurry out again.[7] Alan Brown had no time to bother with bookkeeping — after all, Connie handled all their finances at home, even remembering to give him a quarter on every charity tag day.

Connie's doling out nickles and dimes for Alan's pocket money worked like a charm for many years. He had no need of ready cash. His meals at the hospital were free and at home Connie paid for everything. But one day her system failed. While the Physician-in-Chief was waiting

---

* cabbage = cash

outside the hospital for his chauffeur to bring the car round to the front door to drive him to his afternoon office, a poor man approached him for money. It was not a tag day and Alan Brown's pockets were empty. The beggar would not believe such an impeccably dressed man had no money. Calling him a liar, he angrily knocked the doctor down and ran off as the chauffeur drove up. Tires squealing, William brought the car to a stop and jumped out, reaching down to help his employer to his feet. He dusted him off and soothed his wounded pride. After that episode Connie slipped an emergency quarter into his pocket nearly every day.

Since income tax, imposed during World War I, was supposed to have been temporary, Brown gave little attention to actually paying it. After several years of freedom from inspection, Revenue Canada descended on his office, found the situation not to its liking and fined him. Today such evasion would have cost him the professorship and his position as Physician-in-Chief at the hospital. But in those days he was able to get away with it — twice. After the first time, Grace Haldenby remembers, "he got very fussy and was careful to have the books audited that year. He did strange things like bringing me a handful of dollar bills to put in the desk. He seemed to want to show me he was an honest man." After a while the bookkeeping slipped once more and the tax department descended again. "We knew we had to tighten things up and not let it happen a third time — and it didn't!" Alan Brown was by now convinced that income tax was not a temporary measure as promised and he decided that he might as well learn to live with it.

He had no interest in becoming a wealthy man. Nevertheless, as a matter of professional principle, he would not reduce his fees for anyone that he knew was able to pay them. Mrs. Tamblyn brought her four children to him and suggested that he might look after them all for the price of one. He was not enthusiastic about the proposal and responded in no uncertain terms. The curt rebuff did not end their relationship. Mrs. Tamblyn had merely been trying for a bargain. Other mothers, such as Mrs. Diamond, said she could not pay him because she had to pay her butcher, milkman, greengrocer and her Chinese laundryman, in addition to looking after her great aunt's expenses. Knowing that her financial circumstances were good, he chided her, "Come now, Mrs. D., let's not have any excuses."

On the other hand he refused to accept payment from those whom he knew could ill afford his fees. As one former patient said: "Getting sick in the thirties was a disaster. We had to be in pretty bad shape before Mother took us to the doctor." Alan Brown was well aware of the financial hardship many of his patients were suffering during the Depression and he quite often waived his fees for office visits and even for house calls. He would accept nothing from Sir Wylie Grier's daughter Stella, an artist herself whose husband had left her with two small children and very little else. Grateful but embarrassed by his generosity she approached Mrs. Brown to ask if she thought Dr. Brown would let her repay him by drawing pastel portraits of their daughters. Connie Brown was delighted at the idea and did not hesitate to accept the offer on behalf of her husband.

He had many other patients he did not allow to pay, the children of doctors (the usual custom before medicare) and members of his extended family:

> He looked after grandfather's twenty-one grandchildren and when they were grown up they presented him with a chaise longue. Their timing was providential. That was in the early thirties when he had bursitis and spent the whole summer at his cabin on Ahmic Lake lounging in their reclining chair. He also broke out in boils from time to time. He was unhappy and grumpy most of the summer. When he returned to the city he went to a dentist who removed an infected tooth and that was the end of the bursitis.[8]

Private Practice Rivalry

When Grace Haldenby was asked if the other paediatricians liked him, her tactful answer was, "I think that might be 'iffy'." Alan Brown was wary of his rivals, both on his staff and in the community. He was always on the watch for any "stealing" of his patients. Whether he was right or not, Brown often thought Sandy Goodchild, a rugged individualist and non-conformist, was guilty of "stealing".

— Sandy had a kind of yo-yo existence, bouncing on and off the Sick Kids' staff at the whim of Alan with a regularity that amused the rest of the staff.[9]
— It was really an insult for a patient to leave him because he

was the best in town at that time. If he thought any of his colleagues had taken a patient away from him he'd remove their hospital privileges. Competition for paying patients was fierce. I can remember one of Dad's patients deserting him and we didn't shop at his store afterwards.[10]

Alan Brown pulled no punches in his private practice whether he was bullying the mothers for not following his instructions or belittling other doctors whose patients often came to him for consultation. John Slavens regrets

he had these little tricks. If you had the kid on one thing he'd prescribe the same thing but a different brand. He just had to change something. Because of this pettiness he was sort of cut off when he retired.

In such a situation he insinuated he knew more than his rival. The tragedy was he had no need to practise one-upmanship. He was the best paediatrician in town in his time, but he lacked the self-confidence to co-operate with his paediatric colleagues and gain their friendship in addition to the respect they grudgingly accorded him. Brian Schwartz could have had Brown in mind when he wrote:

Great achievement usually requires a great will to succeed and the near-total application of time and emotional energy . . . . To achieve recognition beyond your competitors, it also helps to be aggressive about grabbing credit — you shove aside collaborators and downgrade your competitors.[11]

Protective of his reputation and jealous of his practice, he would often pretend not to know the referring doctor. After a pause, unsettling to the patient, he would mutter, "Snelling? Snelling? Let me see. Yes, of course, one of my students." Or: "Silverthorne? I taught him everything he knows." Or, "Goodchild, surely he didn't tell you to do *that*?" finishing with the astute conclusion, "How fortunate that you have now come to me." If he disagreed with a colleague's diagnosis or treatment he would never bother to be diplomatic to spare the other's reputation. Nelles Silverthorne, used to "Alan's little tricks", once had the fun of outfoxing him:

I was treating little Peggy Kirkpatrick for chronic diarrhea. Her parents wanted a second opinion so I advised them to go to Alan Brown. He looked through his fluoroscope and said, "Oh, she's got coeliac disease. Put her on protein milk." I'd had her on lactic acid milk and was just about to try protein milk, but I knew that would leave him no avenue to disagree with what I'd done so I left it to him to change the milk. When I told him later, he said with a twinkle in his eye, "Well, I had to try something different didn't I?"

His wife smiled, "That was the only way to handle Alan Brown."

The Infants' Home
Alan Brown was the consultant to the Board of the Infants' Home, now a part of the Childrens' Aid Society. Dr. Helen Reid worked at the Home from 1938 to 1941, "at a time when we locked up the unwed mothers. Brown was adamant that they be kept there to nurse their babies for three months whether or not they were giving them up for adoption. It just wrings my heart to remember the mother's anguish when she had to give her baby up." Laurie Chute responded to his wife's distress, "He was protecting those babies from dying. This is the kind of trade-off medicine is always making. You must judge such things in the context of their times." Helen Reid continued:

> In those days we had an excess of 6000 children waiting for adoption. Many had defects that are now correctable. Alan Brown and all the other paediatricians would not recommend them for adoption when there were so many healthy babies available. We had a beautiful one-year-old with lovely red hair. A young couple wanted to adopt her. Alan inspected the child but advised against adoption. She had an underslung jaw just like the former Toronto mayor! I was upset about his rejection. We arranged through the Children's Aid to send the child to an orthodontist. There was only one in Toronto in those days. He made appliances and a gadget for her when she sucked on her bottle and he eventually fell in love with her and adopted her himself.
>
> By today's standards the medical attitude towards the retarded or

handicapped children was outrageous. But in those days so little could be done for them that Alan Brown and his contemporaries feared the extra attention required for their nurture over the years would adversely affect the stability of the whole family. His philosophy was to let the physically handicapped and mentally retarded babies die as comfortably as possible. Some of his colleagues admit, and Bill Hawke was adamant that

> he'd simply starve them. He'd put them on feedings of one ounce of milk with water. I know that he advised the parents that this should be done. A friend of mine, a doctor, decided to do the same thing with his own child.

One of his senior residents, Dr. Robert Farber, recalls:

Alan Brown was really cruel with parents. I think he was trying to make it clear just how hopeless the future was for these babies. He was trying to save them trudging from doctor to doctor hoping that something could be done. There was one family whose child was born severely brain-damaged. They were a nice, hardworking young couple. Dr. Brown examined their baby and told the parents it was hopeless to hope, but they asked anyway. "What can we do for him?" His stark reply was, "Leave it by the side of a river." After Dr. Brown had left the room I tried to explain: "What Dr. Brown told you is very, very true," I said. "Your baby has severe cerebral palsy. It's unlikely he will ever walk. But, you know, medicine is constantly evolving and maybe someday something will come along to help your child." That was the last I heard of them for some time. A month after I went into practice, they came to my office with their little boy and that afternoon they became my patients. A year later, when the second baby was born the mother telephoned, "Oh, this baby is just fine so we thought we'd go to our GP." When the child was about six months old they phoned me again, "We're worried, something's wrong with our baby." It had the same thing as the first baby but neither had brain damage as we'd originally thought. The condition was a defect of development and had nothing to do with birth injury. This baby was not as severely handicapped as the first, that's why it wasn't recognized earlier.

The father was a carpenter. He built special equipment for the children to sit in. The last I heard from them, the older child was in his late twenties or early thirties in a half-way house and was able, with sign language and so on, to communicate. The younger one was able to walk and go to a special school. You know, they managed.

Chapter 7
Private Life

IN THE EARLY years of their marriage misfortune dogged Connie and Alan Brown. In those days married couples usually did not choose whether or not to have children. They were expected to have them and when they could they did. The Browns were no exception. Their first daughter, Barbara, arrived without incident in 1917. Connie's next two pregnancies ended in grief: first, a still-born, then another son died in infancy. Many years later, in a conversation with Barbara, her father admitted wistfully, "You know my dear, I think it's a good thing I didn't have any sons; I think I might have expected too much of them."

Shortly after Barbara's birth the Browns hired the first of several nannies and moved from the duplex on the corner of Avenue Road and Balmoral Avenue to a house at 423 Avenue Road, at the top of the hill and beside the Victorian gingerbread mansion that now belongs to De La Salle School. The Brown family lived on the floors above the large basement Alan used as an office and shared with another paediatrician, Roy Simpson. Together they furnished the waiting room and the two offices. Both their private practices grew rapidly and in the early twenties, when Dr. Simpson moved his office to his new house on Scholfield Avenue in Rosedale, Alan Brown installed his chauffeur, William, in the room vacated by Roy Simpson.

Barbara was then nearly eight years old. Connie and Alan despaired of having another baby but both wanted to spare their daughter the lone-

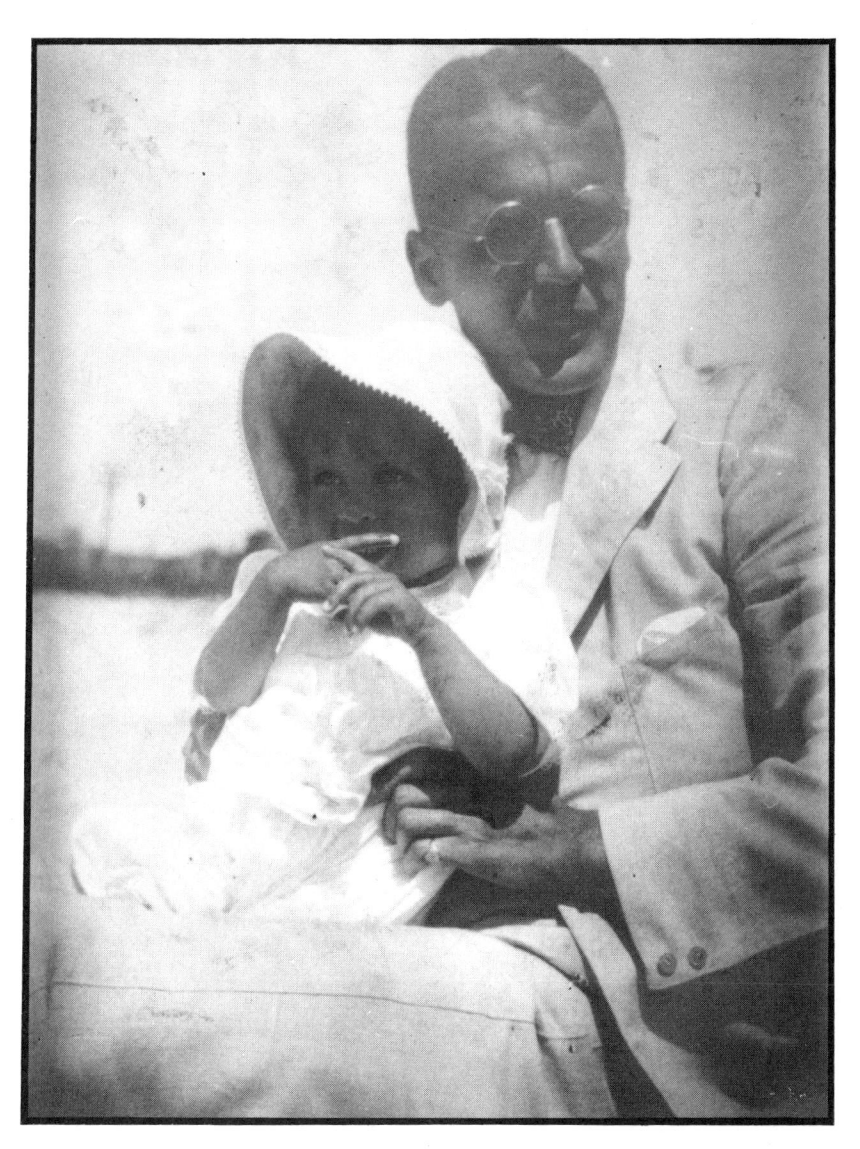

A lap full of Barbara, about 1920

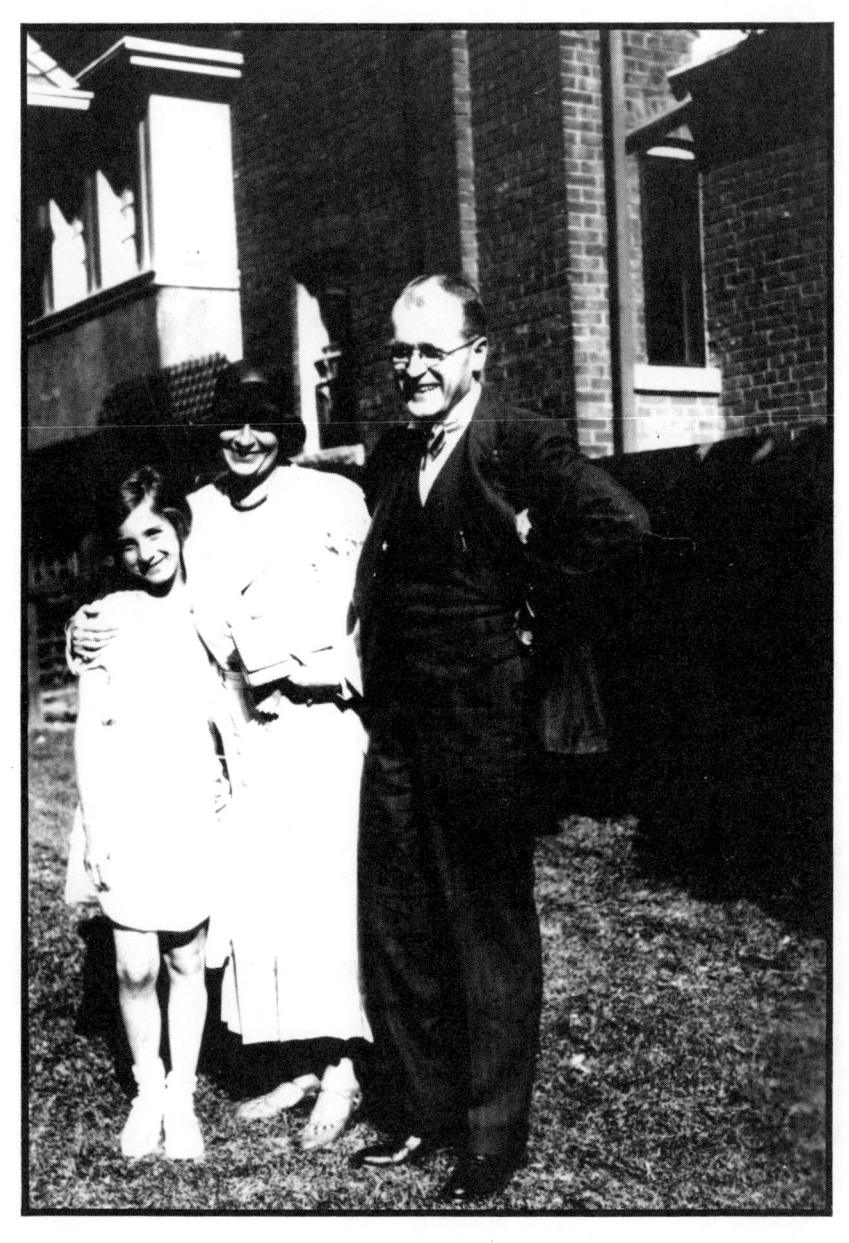

Nancy with parents, about 1933

liness of being an only child. Lady Peacock, a friend of Connie's, proposed that the Browns consider adopting a little girl from an English orphanage endowed by the Peacocks. Alan, who knew how much Connie liked to travel, suggested that she and her sister Tot go off to England to investigate. Nothing loath, away they went and returned with Nancy, aged two. Barbara remembers her excitement when she first saw Nancy: "O God! She was cute!" Her cousin, Tot's daughter Elisabeth, recalls the details:

> Mother and Auntie Conn took turns walking the deck with Nancy. She loved it — nearly wore them out. Uncle Alan couldn't wait to see them and took the train to Montreal to meet the boat. Nancy wore a little blue velvet coat trimmed with white fur, a matching bonnet and tiny black patent leather shoes. On the train, she sat solemnly in the seat opposite him. She was just gorgeous and he sat bug-eyed all the way from Montreal to Toronto.

The two little girls passed their early childhood in the rambling old house that Alan and Connie rented from the sister of R.R. McCormick, the controversial owner and publisher of the *Chicago Tribune*. In those days Miss McCormick owned all the present De La Salle property on Avenue Road and lived in the big old mansion on the crest of the hill. She loved children and adopted a little boy and a little girl — an unusual step for an unmarried woman in those days. (The boy became a doctor and is now practising in the States.) Miss McCormick gave wonderful Christmas parties for all the neighbourhood children. She built a skating rink every winter and in other ways encouraged the children to play in her spacious grounds. One summer evening she gave a grand ball attended by the cream of Toronto society. Barbara and Nancy nearly fell out their bedroom window as they tried to spot their parents strolling under the lanterns hanging from the trees. Through the open windows of the brightly lit mansion the strains of a dance band playing the Charleston drifted across the lawn to fire the imaginations of the two little girls: "Mummy's good at that — I wish we could see her."

Alan, in spite of his experience with children, was surprised to find that the first time he spanked Barbara was more difficult than he expected. She was three or four when he overheard her shouting rudely at her nanny. Such behaviour was in defiance of his own consideration and respect for servants. He grabbed his squirming daughter, slung her over his knees and spanked her. Long afterwards he told her, "It was too much for me. When I set you on your feet again, your bonnet had fallen over your face and you were crying bitterly. That finished me. I told your mother, never again" — a promise he was unable to keep.

One cold winter day Barbara was terrified she would get the hairbrush treatment. She had been playing with the neighbourhood children on the skating rink when

> Pete McCurdy turned the hose on me and I ran home soaked, my clothes crackling as they froze. Nobody came when I hammered on the door crying my eyes out so I ran down to Dad's door, scared to disturb him, but my teeth were chattering I was so cold. The patients looked up as I burst into his office. He took one look, handed me his key and said, "Get up to your room and get out of your wet clothes" — and that was the end of it. I couldn't believe I'd escaped so easily.

Alan and Connie Brown had difficulty adjusting to their new parental roles, partly because neither had a sensitive nature. But over the years both learned to be understanding, in a blinkered sort of way, when the situation cried out loudly enough to gain their attention. Neither Alan nor Connie had had warm and loving mothers, and their fathers' daily absences at business had offered few opportunities to develop close relationships. Connie was indifferent to the motherly role expected of her. She loved Barbara and Nancy in an offhand way. She liked them to be polite and look pretty and was proud of their accomplishments. She was more affectionate than her own aloof mother who had almost ignored her children, finding them tiresome distractions from her formal social life. By contrast, Connie was less of a slave to social conventions as she moved easily within the structured society of that time.

> In the old days there were always old aunts to visit or take for a drive. She went out for lunch a lot to places like the Ladies Club and she played mah jong like mad. She may have had bridge parties but she didn't play. And in those days you always had people in for tea. But her passion was antiques. There wasn't an antique shop in Toronto that didn't know her.[1]

Connie Brown collected porcelain, lovely old silver and antique furniture, especially mahogany and old oak. She would keep her purchases hidden until it was too late to take them back and then she would slyly bring them out. Her husband would roll his eyes to the ceiling: "Conn, where *did* you get that?" She often went to England with her sister Tot and two or three friends "and they always came back loaded."

Alan Brown's love and concern for children in general is well known, but his life as a busy paediatrician left him little time to foster a close relationship with his own. Affectionate and teasing, or bad-tempered and stern, he was always natural with his patients but self-conscious with his own young daughters. In his professional role he was always sure of himself but in his domestic persona he was fuzzy and uncertain. At home he was simply out of his element.

Confrontations with Nancy he found difficult. He recognized that she was much like himself — stubborn, proud, on guard, aggressive. He respected her independent thinking but didn't know how to handle her when they clashed. Nor could he express his affection other than mutter his pet name for her — Tiny — to show the depth of his feelings. He could tease Barbara with whom he felt more at ease, but not Nancy.

Barbara and her mother were cheerful chatterboxes. Alan just sat back and listened to their thoughts skipping into their minds and out again almost before they knew what they were saying. Connie was usually so caught up in her story of the moment that she was unaware of his chuckle, while an attentive twinkle in his eye was the only response Barbara ever expected. She was never wary or fearful of his reactions to her confidences or her activities.

Barbara did not matriculate from high school. "My reports used to be horrendous. Dad would groan, then laugh. 'Money down the drain. But, you've done your best and that's what counts.'" He knew she loved him, and she would accept his judgement without question. They could relax in each other's company.

Nancy resembled her adoptive father, determined to have her own way and to keep any show of affection under wraps. "I know he loved me but he couldn't show it. He was scared of being hurt. He built a wall so high people couldn't get close to him. I've done that too."

In the early twenties the Browns added a Chinese cook to the household, a fashionable acquisition at the time. His name had been anglicized to George. Barbara and Nancy did not often resist the temptation to tease him:

> We had a parrot we used to swing back and forth on an old bedsheet in the attic playroom. Polly loved it and she'd squawk, "More, more." Her cage was at the top of the stairs and William the chauffeur used to pop up to stroke her feathers and Polly would purr — just like a cat. Nancy had taught her to say, "Damn Dr. Brown."

The morning they let Polly out of the cage she preened herself quietly on top of the door frame. George arrived to fetch their breakfast tray:

> He didn't notice the cage was empty. When he left, Polly took off after the shiny bald head descending the stairs. A terrified George threw his hands up for protection and the tray went flying. Poor George, he nearly broke his neck sliding down the stairs.

The excitement was too much for Polly who repeatedly squawked, "Damn Dr. Brown, damn Dr. Brown":

> The commotion disturbed Dad. When he came up "to find out what the hell was going on," I got such a walloping. Polly was given to the chauffeur's wife and from then on every time I got spanked, the parrot would say, "poor Nancy, poor Nancy".

Nancy always stood her ground, daring Alan to punish her:

> He used to spank with his carpet slipper. Once when I was mad at mother I went into the huge cupboard where she did her household accounts. I found a shoe box full of old letters and pictures and I attacked the lot, not really knowing their significance. It was great fun to tear them all up. When Dad found out — I didn't sit down for a week.

Even when Nancy infuriated him he could be amused, however reluctantly. He had a grudging respect for the defiance by which she tried to justify her behaviour, just as he respected those who defied him with good reason at the hospital.

By 1927 the Browns had outgrown their rented house on the Avenue Road hill. Alan Brown moved his office up to 217 St. Clair Avenue West and bought a house close by at 51 Dunvegan Road. During most of the twenty years the Browns lived there they employed the same cook and housemaid:

> We just adored Annie and Norah. They were an important part of our family, specially since mother couldn't cook and was terrified of the Hoover. When the maids weren't there they left something cold for supper and we all had to pile in and do the dishes. Even Dad would help dry if he wasn't out making a call. Mother was great with the household accounts, ingenious as a decorator but hopeless in the kitchen. Father used to laugh, "Conn's the only one I know who can burn water."

Connie and her sisters never learned to cook. The maids the Hobbs employed did not permit interference in "their" kitchen. Alan, however, had grown up without such constraints that affluence imposed and rather liked "to do a little mashing around with a frying pan."

While the Browns were a united family in the sense of presenting one face to the world, they didn't communicate well with one another. For example, nobody warned Nancy whenever she was to have an operation. One morning as she came down to breakfast the telephone was ringing, but since Annie and Norah were in the kitchen she answered it herself. After the caller had confirmed that it was Dr. Brown's house she continued with her message: "We're expecting the little girl at the hospital tomorrow." Since Barbara was away at boarding school there was only one little girl left in the house. Alarmed, Nancy hung up and ran to Annie and Norah: "Am I going to the hospital?" They looked at each other. "Yes, Miss Nancy. You're to have your appendix out." To relieve his guilt for leaving Nancy to find out in such a way, Alan had a surprise for her when she came home from the hospital:

> This is something I remember, very fondly. Dad came up the stairs to the attic and he had a little Pekinese in his hand. He peeked around the door — you know, with the bow tie and

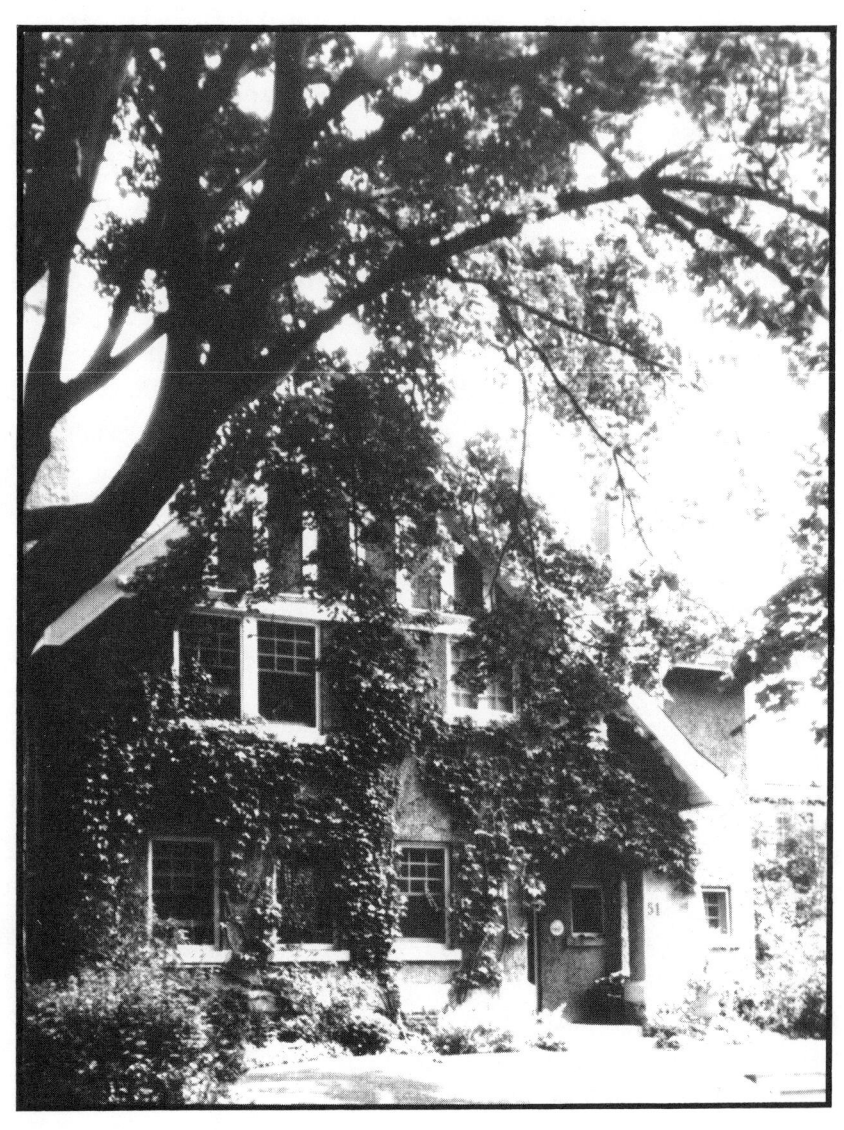

51 Dunvegan Road, Toronto

looking over his glasses. "I have a present for you." And he put a little dog on my bed, so small it suited my nickname, so we called her Tiny. From then on we always had a pair of Pekes.

Alan thought every child should have a dog. "It teaches them to be kind," he said.

First, there was an Airedale called Bobs. I can just remember him, so I must have been about five. Someone let him out on to Avenue Road and a car hit him. Dad and Mother were heartbroken. Then we had a mutt called Mickey Moo who used to walk beside Nancy as she was pushed along in her old wicker stroller. We got into Pekes because father looked after the McCarthy family. That's where Nancy's puppy came from. Their house is now part of Branksome Hall School.

Summers along the Magnetawan
By the spring of 1929, when he was forty-two years old, the pressure of Alan Brown's increasing responsibilities and success finally began to reflect on his health and he bowed to the wisdom of his cardiologist colleague Dr. John Oille. Oille's prescription: two-months holiday every summer. Alan promptly rented a cottage at Kennebunk Beach in Maine.

Before he left the city with his family at the end of June he spoke to Nelles Silverthorne: "Silver, I want you to take my summer practice. You're on call twenty-four hours a day till the beginning of September. Don't let me down !" Alan Brown's summer office became a lasting responsibility for the ever-willing Dr. Silverthorne.

There was more adventure in the drive down and back than there was in the golf courses and the sands of Kennebunk Beach. The Browns drove a marvel of automotive engineering, an old Franklin convertible with a canvas roof so high the ladies could climb in and out without knocking their hats askew. In deference to the danger of losing them at the top speed of twenty or twenty-five miles per hour, they wound veils over the hats tying them securely at the neck.

Maine was a long drive over washboard gravel roads that spewed dust and blew out a tire almost every hour. Alan Brown soon wearied of the annual trek. When, in 1932, his friend and colleague, D.E. Robertson, told him about a cottage for sale near the village of Magnetawan,

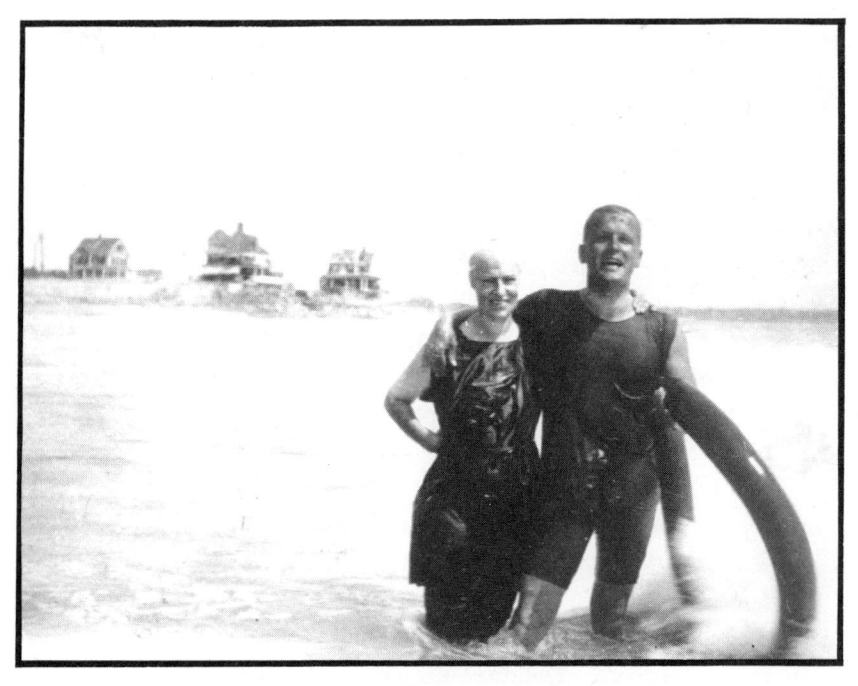

Alan and Connie at Kennebunk Beach, 1921

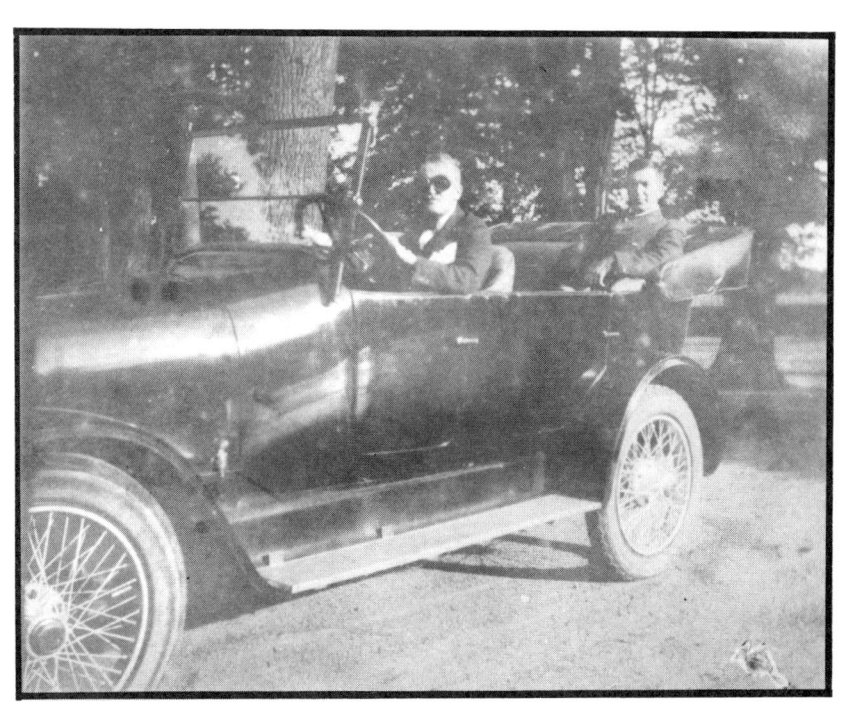

Alan at the wheel of his touring car, 1921

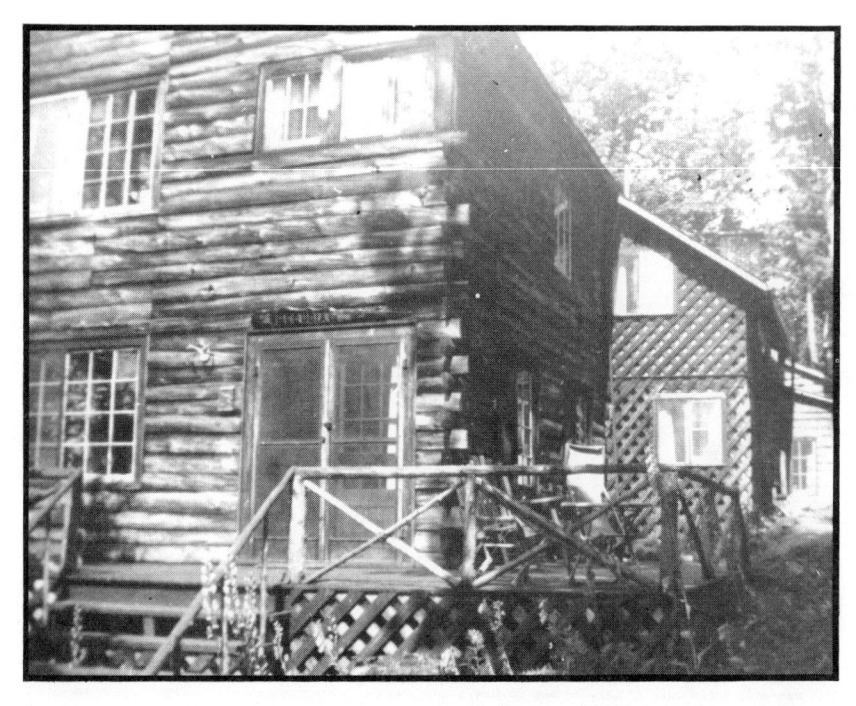

"Sequoia", home of Alan's other life

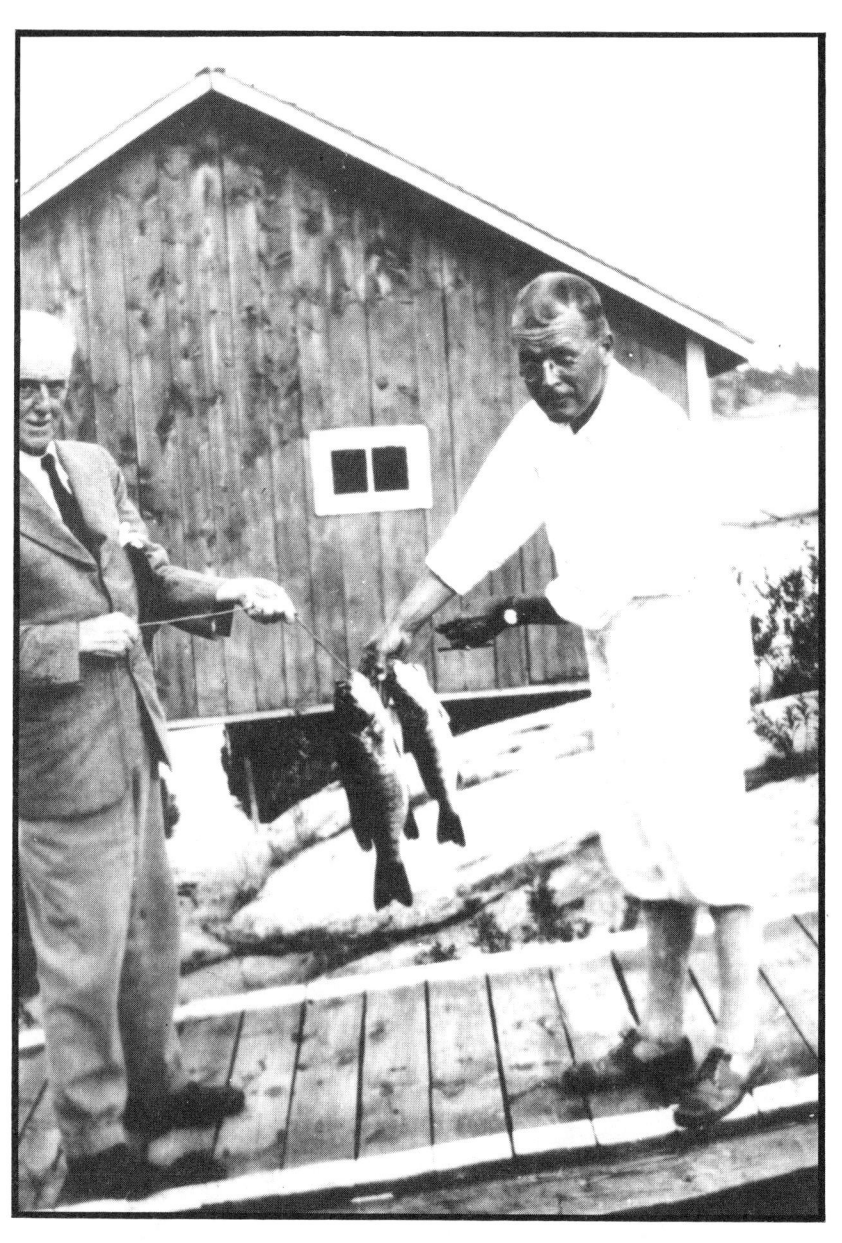

Fillets for supper from Grant Fisher and Alan Brown

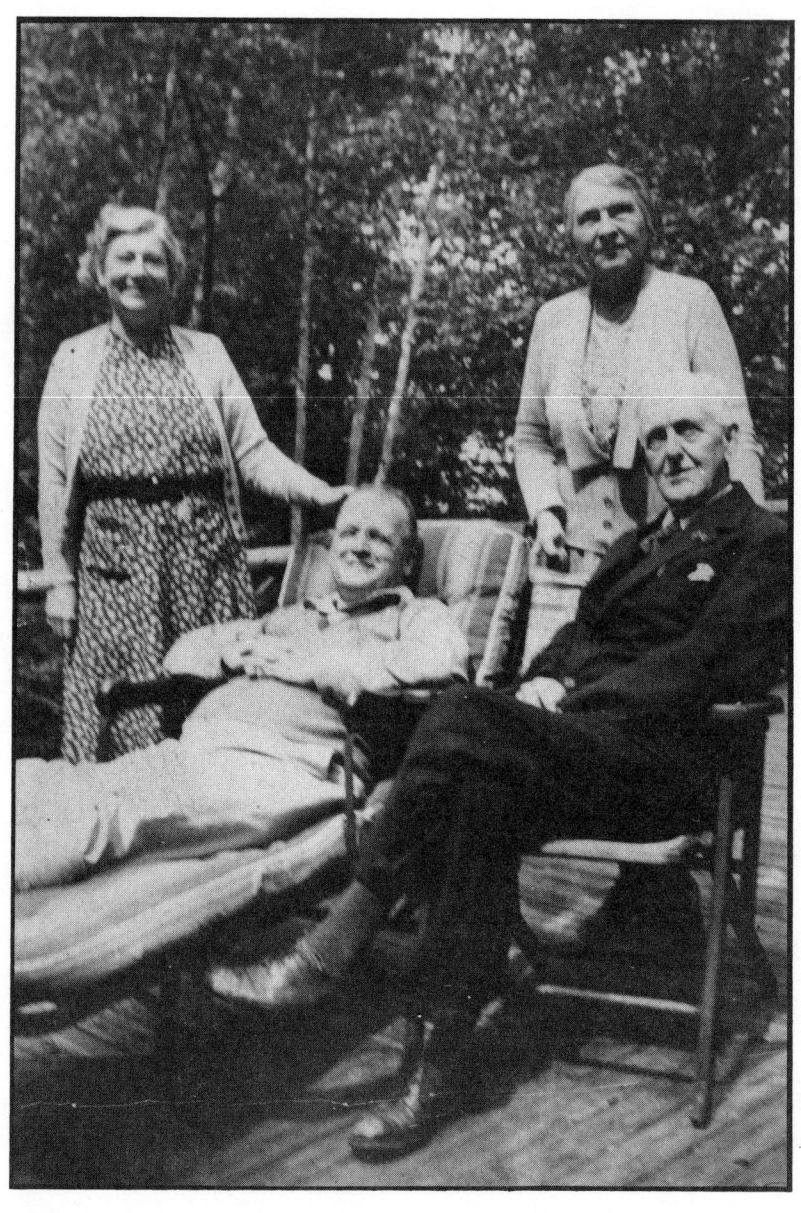

Alan Brown and Grant Fisher hobnobbing with Connie and Tot at "Sequoia" in the late 1930s

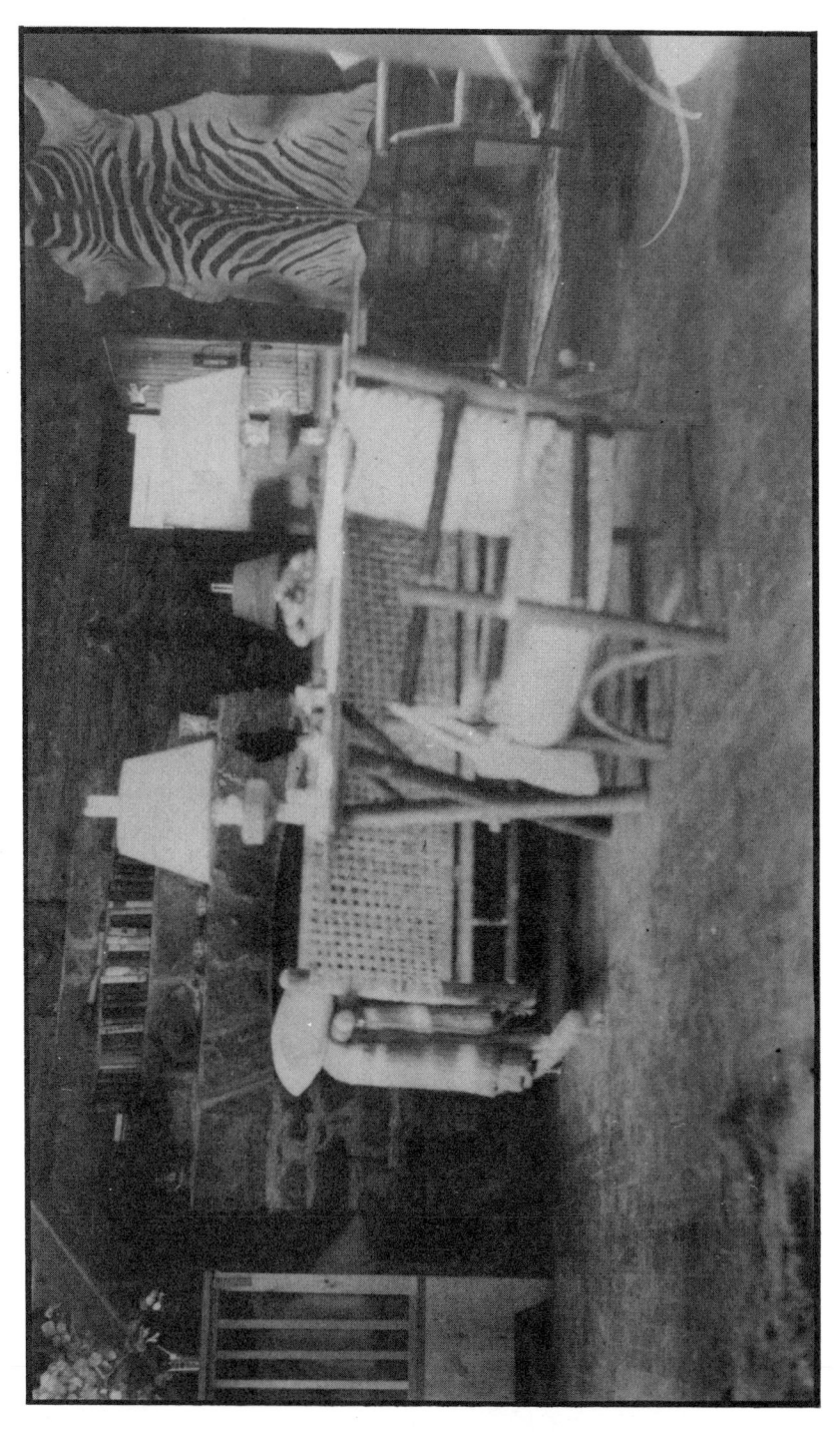

Cabin's living room displays Alan's skill in carpentry

the Browns snapped it up. Compared to Maine it was an easy drive from Toronto, but still far enough away from the demands of hospital and patients. The clapboard and log cabin on Ahmic Lake not far from the mouth of the Magnetawan River was ideal. During the next twenty years at the cabin Alan named "Sequoia", the Browns built many memories to share for the rest of their lives.

There were *cabins* and *cottages* on Ahmic Lake. To Alan Brown, log cabins were far superior to wood-frame cottages no matter how grand they were. The Browns' cabin looked north across the lake so that in late August they could often watch the Northern Lights flashing against the night sky. The main building was made of stripped cedar logs. A frame addition faced with board and batten stained to blend with the old logs completed the dwelling. Its two storeys had enough rooms to accommodate the family, the beloved and indispensable Annie and Norah and weekend guests. Connie's female relatives often came with their husbands and over the years became close friends of the Browns. Alan rarely saw members of his own family. He was fond of his father but was not prepared to suffer his mother's constant carping. Connie's family and his mother's sisters, Grace and Susan Gowans, filled his need for a congenial domestic life. He basked in the admiration of his maternal aunts and had many interests in common with his sisters-in-law and their husbands. Each spring he would tease Connie with, "What kind of harem will I have this summer?"

Inside the cabin there was a huge stone fireplace, pine furniture, and chairs covered in a weave of soft colours in yellow and orange. On the old polished pine floor lay an oval braided rug worked in warm beige with brown flecks. Scattered around it were several fur rugs and on the wall to the right of the fireplace hung a zebra skin. Comfortably cushioned wooden chairs with wide arms gave evidence of Alan's carpentry skills. Green, almost translucent curtains hung on the generous windows overlooking the lake and the grounds which Alan attacked sporadically with scythe and hatchet, eager to battle them into submission. Outside, on a weathered board above the French doors leading into the living room, he had carved "Sequoia". A verandah ran across the front and down one side of the building. Below the verandah, along its entire length, Connie planted nasturtiums, lupins, Canterbury bells and ferns.

Sequoia's previous owner — the Browns named her Auntie Matt — had left behind a lot of odds and ends of clothes. One day Alan found her old bathing suit of black silk with a knee-length skirt and put it on. Adding a straw hat tied with a green ribbon under his chin and carrying a purple parasol he swaggered down to the dock under the eyes of six women, a captive audience for his antics. He walked to the end of the diving board holding his nose, the parasol raised, and jumped into the lake. To the delight of the spectators the skirt flew up as he flew down. He had nothing on underneath. "He often acted without thinking. He liked to play the fool and make us laugh."

When her father bought a sailboat Barbara abandoned Miss Case's camp for girls to spend her summers at Sequoia. She sailed in the weekly races with Alan or Uncle Billy Woods [2] as her crew. One year Barbara and her father won the sailing trophy. The next season they raised a bright orange sail that he had brought back from Scotland to replace the white one which he said was "dull and boring" — a gesture typical of his independent spirit.

Connie and Alan swam every day in every kind of weather. He loved to fish and to play horseshoes with his family and friends. He chortled with glee when he won and was good-humoured if he lost. When he went up the lake for the mail he would spend a lazy hour chatting with the Rafflaubs, the local family who owned the marina at Magnetawan. As a teenager, Thelma Rafflaub worked for the Browns in the summer. The association turned her ambition towards a nursing career, but she had not yet passed high school matriculation, the minimum entrance requirement. One day Thelma arrived at the Browns' in tears.

> Mother hurried into the living room where Dad was quietly reading. "Alan, Thelma is crying her eyes out!" "Why?" "She's just got her matric results and she's flunked history." "History!" Father snorted. "What's that got to do with nursing? Well, history of a patient, yes, but HISTORY?" He rushed out to the kitchen, "Don't you worry my dear, I'll fix it up." He jumped into his boat and zoomed to the village where he 'phoned Jean Masten, Director of Nursing at HSC. Thelma was accepted as a probationer and turned out to be one of the best students Sick Kids' ever had.

Paediatric colleagues visiting the Browns at Magnetawan discovered a man no longer threatened by the pressures and competition of profes-

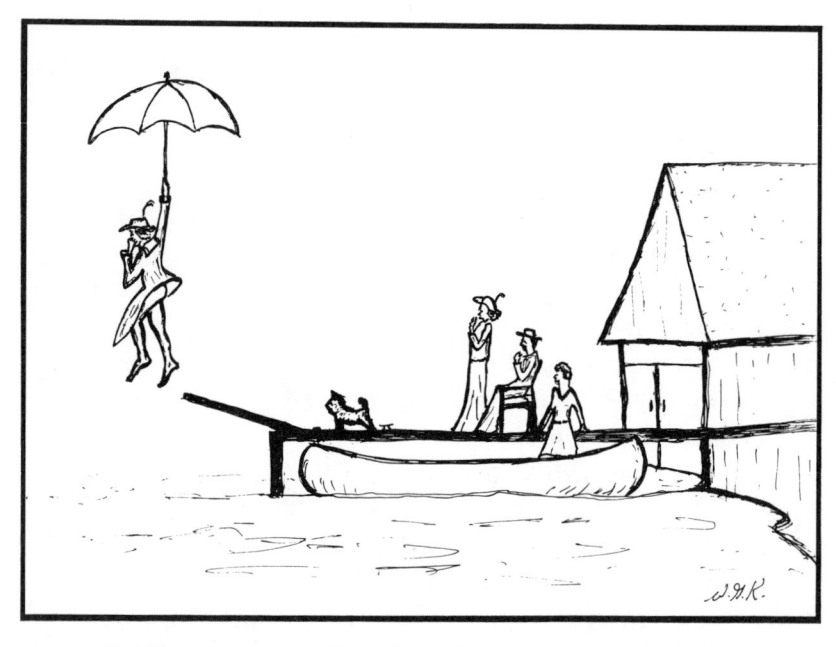

Double exposure — Alan's leap of faith (cartoon by W.G.K.)

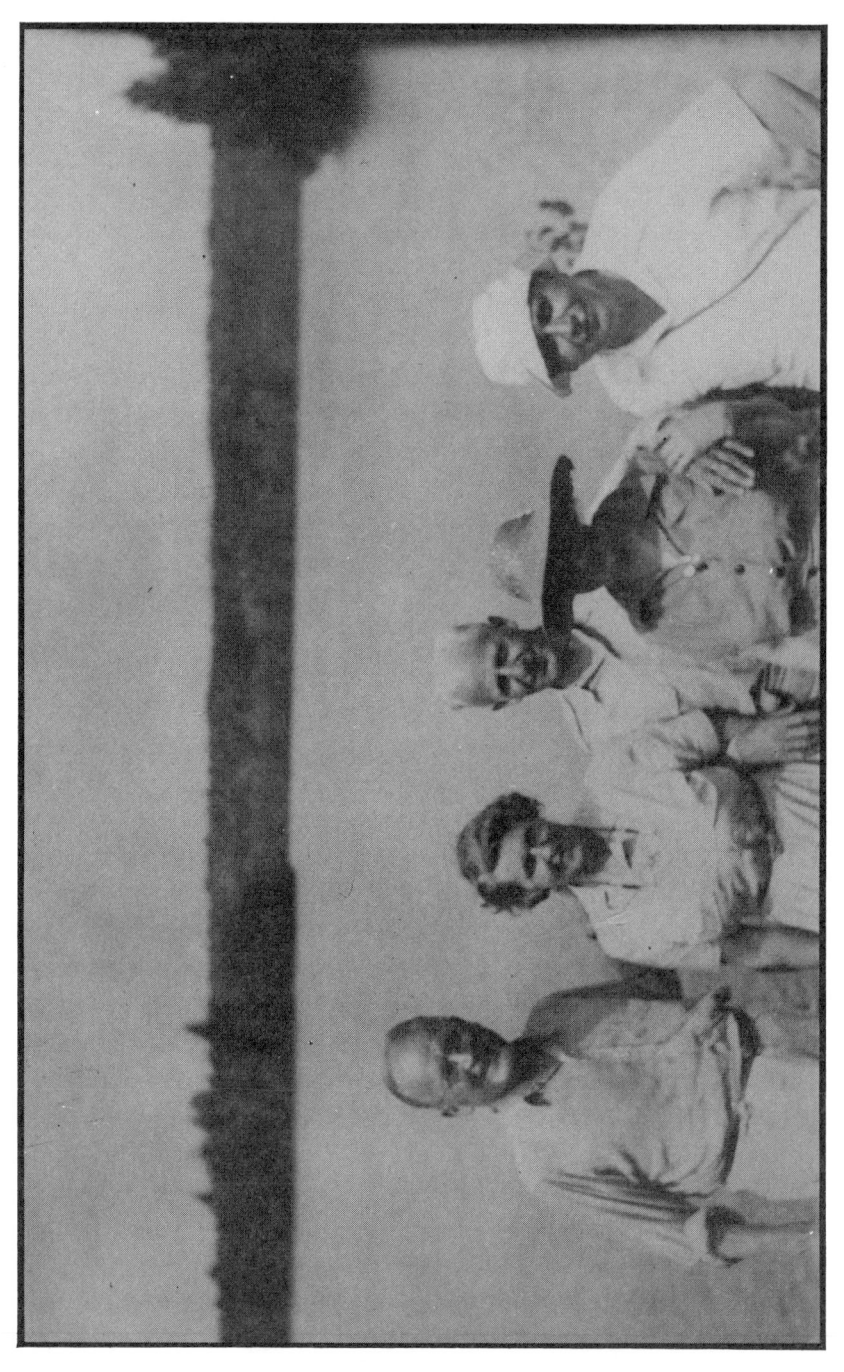

Alan at Ahmic Lake with Clara and Paul Mills of Toronto, Connie and Ben Merritt, professor of classics at Princeton, 1951

sional life. Alan was friendly, amusing and relaxed, but he couldn't entirely shed the image of a healer: he was in great demand as a veterinarian. He set the broken limbs of neighbours' pets and removed porcupine quills from the snouts of local dogs. For this operation he subdued the patient into unconsciousness with a spray of ethyl chloride, clipped the ends of the quills to let the air out and then gently withdrew them. His black medical bag was always at the ready for human patients too.

> Dad was forever saying, "Children, look after your fish hooks — don't leave them lying around on the dock." Nancy and I would just roll our eyes. Now Uncle Billy and Auntie Ber (Woods) used to stay with us every summer. Dad and Uncle Billy often went off fishing. One day, Auntie Ber, mother and I were in the living room playing rummy when they returned, Father looking very sheepish. Uncle Billy started to laugh. Father had cast his hook into the back of Uncle Billy's head and he had had to stitch it up.

Alan was a ruthless hunter of the red squirrels that played havoc with the beds and stuffed furniture during the winter. He had an ally in Nancy's Pekinese:

> He took his cue from Tiny. His .22 hung on the wall in the living room just inside the screen doors. Tiny would scratch on the door, jumping up and down and then rush to the verandah railing. The cabin was up high with a lovely view of the lake through the trees. Father understood. When she saw him take his rifle down, she'd go mad, tearing down the steps. Down below she would look up at the tree where the squirrel had taken refuge. Dad would shoot it and Tiny would retrieve the body once it had fallen to earth, dash up the stairs and lay it at his feet.

In the autumn he hunted partridge but Tiny stayed at home with the family. One year Harry and Couchi Ebbs were invited when the season opened. It was one of those dreamy warm Thanksgivings when the sun brought out the full glory of the forest. The Ebbs arrived to find Alan in shorts, bare to the waist, bailing out the sailboat: "It was one of the most informal weekends we ever had. Connie was wonderful, unconventional as always. She made Alan approachable."

In a time of severe anxiety, Mary Tisdall found true friends in the Browns. Fred, Mary's husband, was in the Arctic to survey the nutritional state of the native population when his 'plane went down. During the four-day search for the missing 'plane, the Browns kept Mary at Sequoia with them until the news came through that the aircraft and its three uninjured occupants had been found.

Alan invited Nelles Silverthorne on another Thanksgiving weekend. Nelles was not in favour of disturbing nature's tranquillity nor destroying the lives of birds with gun shot:

> Alan asked me up north on a shooting expedition, for partridge or whatever those birds are called. I saw him take just an ordinary — what do you call those guns, shotguns, rifles? — and pick the bird right out of the air — amazing — while it was flying. Well, they took me along. Two of his brothers-in-law and Ted Morgan were there, and all of them crack shots. Alan turned to me and said, "Now, there's one right down there just waiting for you." Why, I could have blown it right off the face of the earth. Maybe I did. I took a shot at it and then it was gone. "Oh," he said, disappointed, "That's too bad," and he patted me on the back. There was so much shooting I thought the Third World War had started.

At the end of the day they would all sit around the fire with their drinks and exchange hunting and fishing tales departing farther and farther from the truth as the evening wore on.

Waving the Star-Spangled Banner
In the 1930s Johns Hopkins was probably the best known of all the medical schools in North America and three or four of its top professors had cottages on Ahmic Lake. Their proximity had been an incentive for the Browns to buy Auntie Matt's cottage. "A bit of a snob", Alan Brown liked the idea of summering among his distinguished peers, and for Connie their neighbours' social status was well up to standard.

> We had some interesting people up there. One was Dr. Flexner. He brought Einstein out to the School for Advanced Studies at Princeton. Abraham Flexner was adorable, a tiny little man

with a hooked nose and married to a Christian. I stayed with them when I visited Princeton. One summer at the lake he and his wife had a guest from Britain. This man looked like a cartoon, wore a pith helmet and World War I army shorts. They were very wide and didn't cover his bony knees. He really was a sight. One day I took my four-year-old, Ann, to the village to get the post. When she saw this creature on the dock beside Dr. Flexner she didn't notice his funny clothes — only his helmet. In a shrill voice she asked him, "Why have you got a pee pot on your head?" When Dad heard the story he laughed till he cried.[3]

Ahmic Lake was full of Americans. "They used to call *us* the foreigners!" Nancy remembers they came from Baltimore, Kentucky, Pittsburgh. Some were professors from Massachusetts Institute of Technology, Princeton and Columbia. The Canadians included the Chesters who, with the Iveys from London, and the D.E. Robertsons, took turns holidaying in the same cottage. Many log cabin owners were also American: Senator Swager Shirley from Kentucky, Mrs. Oliver from Baltimore and several from Pittsburgh, such as Mrs. Lloyd, "a lovely old lady". And then there was Dr. Kelley, a founder of Johns Hopkins and a pompous old bore who rode herd on his many great-grandchildren and their parents who were all bullied into spending their holidays in the many cabins on his large property:

He was an awful old crab and far too straight-laced for Dad who'd groan, "Conn, do we have to go in to church today? Howard is going to speak." Once Dr. Kelley interrupted his sermon, leaned over the pulpit and barked a question at one of his mortified grandchildren. Mother and Father were furious.

Alan Brown's days at the cottage were almost as full as in the city. He still devoted most of his evenings to reading, but instead of medical journals he relaxed with novels by G.A. Henty, Edgar Rice Burroughs or Agatha Christie. When the weather was fine, fishing, sailing, canoeing, swimming, hunting and horseshoes captured his full attention. On rainy days he became a jack-of-all-trades, a competent and sometimes inspired carpenter constructing tables, chairs and even beds for his log cabin.

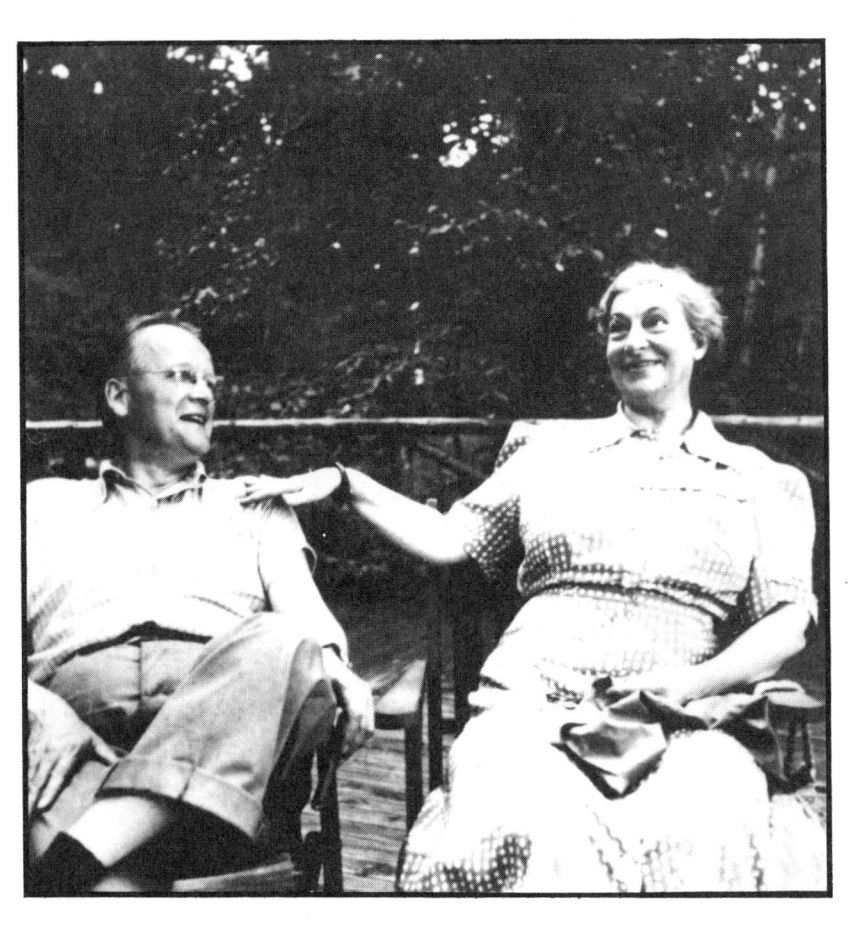

Fred Tisdall snaps Alan and Connie at "Sequoia", July 1940

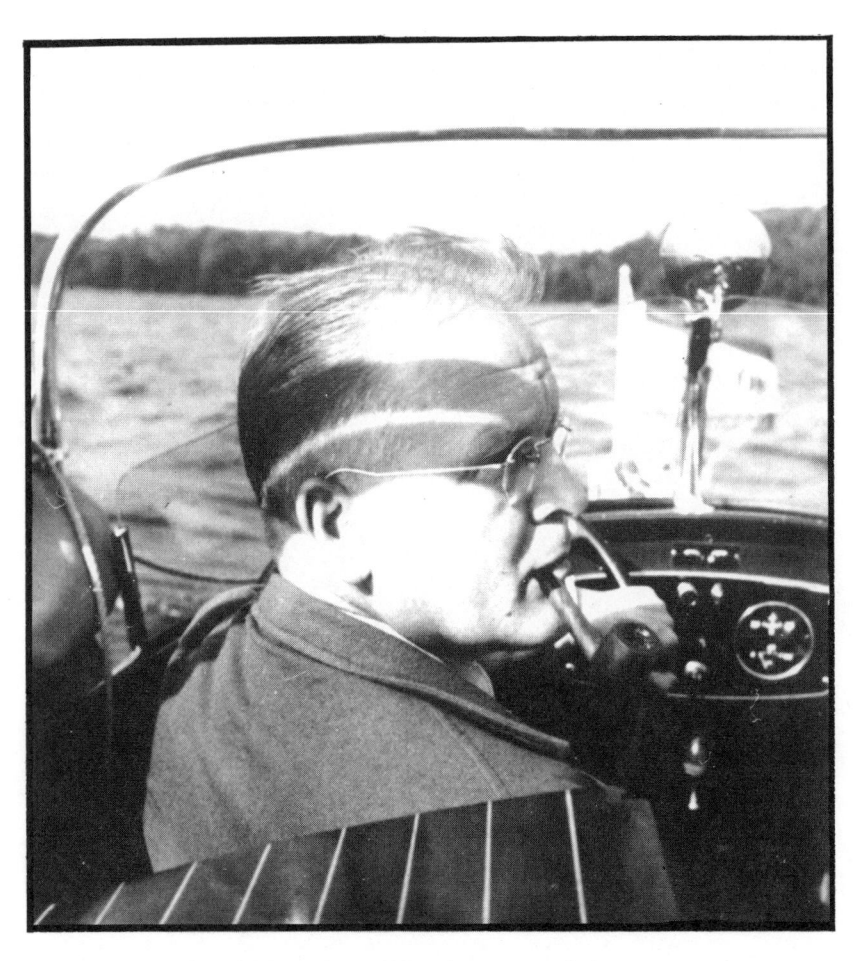

Alan driving the "AlCon", pennant flying, 1941

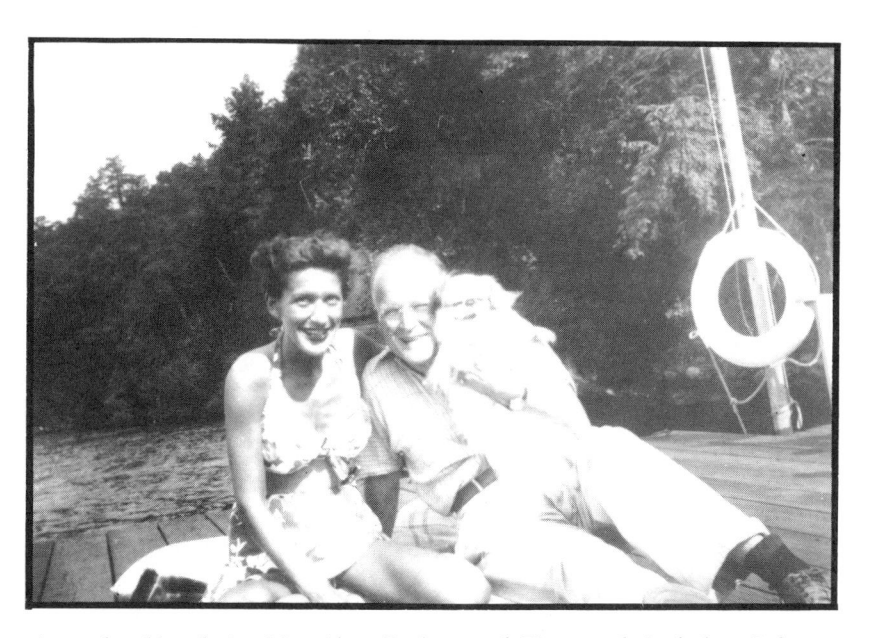

A comfortable relationship: Alan, Barbara and Tiny on their dock at Lake Ahmic, 1943

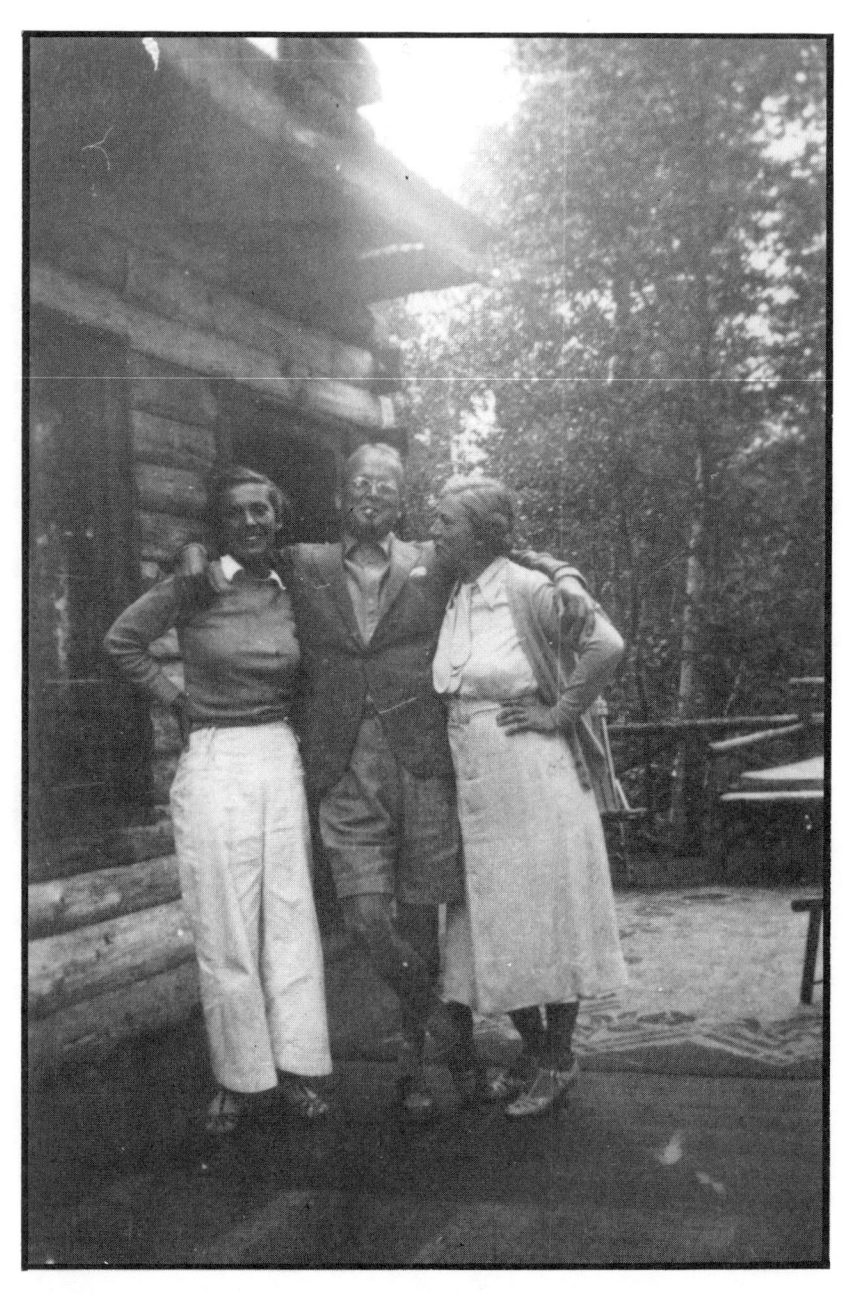

Barbara, Alan and Connie pose on "Sequoia"'s verandah, 1943

He even became a passable plumber. When Connie's teeth fell down the drain into the septic tank he took up the challenge.

"It's the worst thing I've ever fished for," he said as he came up with the captured teeth. I'll never forget him leaning over that tank and stirring it all up with his hands while the rest of us stood well back and watched.

Not long after, Connie's Aunt Sarah Osborne died. With her share of the small estate Connie approached Alan with a sly smile, "Why don't we use some of the money for a proper bathroom?" Her husband needed no persuasion and they laughed as they recalled the amusing problems of the early days at the cabin when they were reading and trying to follow Chic Sale's directions for building a privy.[4] Modern plumbing now had a certain appeal.

In the early mornings or as the sun was setting Alan delighted in canoeing alone along the still waters of the lake or the river. Fishing was his favourite sport. It satisfied his competitive streak to feel the strike and land the fish. He always needed an opponent or a goal. The cleaning of the fish in the boathouse appealed to his sense of order and responsibility. He not only wanted to spare Annie the mess but he was certain that she would not fillet them as well as he. Perfect technique in sport fishing was more important to him than the actual catch. One day Barbara and her husband Bill were fishing from the canoe. Along came her parents and an uncle and aunt in "AlCon", the splendid mahogany motor launch, Alan's pride:

Dad drove up close to us. Bill had hooked a fish. Dad called out, "Play it Bill, play it!" Bill couldn't be bothered, so he just gave a mighty heave with his rod and landed a big bass in the bottom of the canoe — the only fish anyone caught that day. Father laughed, "That will teach me to interfere!"

He didn't take his own advice to heart. Whenever he saw Barbara and Nancy approaching the dock in the boat he had given them he would stand beside the slip and watch them motoring slowly in. There was not much room on either side. Often there was a crosswind which had to be gauged perfectly to prevent bumping. He would watch the landing up to the last moment. Everything had to be done his way.

Bill Kelley was very much at ease with his father-in-law and knew how to handle him. One summer Alan Brown asked him to fix the loose uprights between the posts of the railing on the cabin verandah. Bill began the work to a barrage from Alan of unwanted advice. It wasn't until Bill threatened to hand over the job to his father-in-law that Alan turned away, laughing, and disappeared down the garden.

His niece, Elisabeth Fisher Lawson, remembers him for his friendship and his sense of humour. She was a willing guest at the cottage in the summers before World War II. Together they cut underbrush or stained a piece of furniture he had just crafted. He lost himself in the concentration of working with wood. His creations, as you might expect, were good — attractive yet sturdy. He loved cutting and carving wood but he always wore protective gloves when he was working around the cabin because, as he explained, "My hands tell me what's wrong with my patients."

Not all the memories of Alan Brown at the cottage were tranquil. He had a quick sense of humour but also a terrible temper. Connie and Alan used to have a few noisy fights up at the cabin. Once after he had tripped over a pair of a guest's shoes lying in the middle of the verandah, he blew up at Barbara. Nancy, who was thirteen or fourteen, came to her sister's defence: "How dare you speak to Barbara like that! It's not her fault." He roared back, "Go to your room and mind your own business." All the same, good humour and fun filled his life at the cabin in contrast to the unyielding front of dignity and discipline he presented to the staff at the hospital.

Once a summer those hopeful Thespians, Alan Brown and Grant Fisher, would put on a show.

> Uncle Grant and Dad had a yearly ritual. Aunt Tot and Mother would roll their eyes and groan when they realized what was coming as they watched their husbands go off through the swinging Dutch doors leading from the living room into the dining room. There they lapped up beer, cheese, green onions, and I forget what else. We'd hear them singing and laughing and after a while they'd come back pretending they were absolutely soused. They'd be singing, off-key, and slurring their words. We'd listen to their rendition of "Yo ho ho and a bottle of rum" and other sea shanties such as

> *My father* (hick) *wa' the keeper of the Eddystone Light*
> *An' he married a* (hick) *mermaid there one night.*
> *Out of thish match came offsprings three,* (hick)
> *Two were fishes* (burp) *an' the other was me.*

The rest was unintelligible. They really were funny. Fishing hats askew, they came rolling into the living room, crashing through the Dutch doors and making enough noise to scare any wildlife away for the rest of the night.

Sometimes getting to the cottage was half the thrill:

> Dad had a maroon Lincoln Zephyr. One Saturday in the spring he asked, "Do you want to come to the lake with me?" I said, "Sure." We had to leave at five o'clock in the morning to get up and down the same day. It was more than four hundred miles there and back, mainly on dirt roads. Opposite the Orillia mental hospital he said with a glint in his eye, "I'm going to let her rip." He stomped on the accelerator and away we flew, over ninety miles an hour. There was no traffic at that hour but a crow crashed into the windshield. Fortunately the glass didn't break, but the poor crow did. Dad said, "Dont you ever tell your mother I was going at that speed."

He was wary of his wife's sharp tongue and dodged it if he could.

And then there was Connie

Connie too was a stubborn character accustomed to having her own way. At home she was the boss. She was every bit as strong-willed as he was. To anyone unaware that Connie ruled the roost it would come as a surprise that a spirit so free and unconventional would put up with such an irritating and demanding man as Grace Haldenby described Alan. Over the thirty years as his secretary she also came to know Connie Brown well:

> She was an oddball. A funny looking woman to start with — didn't care what she wore — came to the office in anything that was handy — most unlike him. She was a natterer and absolutely uninhibited. You couldn't help but like her. Just as blunt

and stubborn as he was but much more human. He was the perfect little man — I mean, he thought he was perfect. When Doris was living at the house she'd hear Mrs. Brown warn, "Watch out. Alan's in a helluva mood." She knew how to handle him.

Some acquaintances sniffed at Connie's social pretensions but others were amused by her quick wit. "Yes, she was a snob but she had a keen sense of humour and that's what I liked." Devoid of inhibitions and completely unselfconscious, she entertained with her irreverent comments on anything that popped into her head. "She was a chatterbox — about anything and everything; not intellectual but certainly not stupid. And very likeable."

Her family delighted in her running commentaries:

Mother knew everyone. We'd be dawdling along in her little green Durant. I'd say, "Mother, let's go," but she'd continue her non-stop gossip as we drove past the houses of the people she knew. She had us in stitches: "My dear Mr. Smith lived there — couldn't stand his wife so jumped out the window in '29;" or "Mrs. Whatsit ran out of gas — in her nightgown — silly woman — what a fuss she made." When she mimicked Perkins Bull, waggling her wattles, we all had a fit of the giggles until Dad cried, "Stop, stop," and wiped his eyes. She should have been on the stage. She was very witty and could imitate anybody.

Even in dress their styles differed. He always looked immaculate, but she rarely did. Connie dressed smartly when she had to, but she wasn't interested in women's fashions. Nor was she particularly interested in how her daughters dressed. She asked her niece to help Barbara choose her wardrobe for the debutant parties in the "silly season". And it was Elisabeth again, several years later, who helped buy Barbara's trousseau and bridesmaids' dresses for her wedding.

Connie Brown was always interested in the lives of the tradesmen where she dealt. She was their friend and knew everything that was going on in their families. She was an extrovert deriving contentment from the kindness and attention she gave to others. Her husband, at the personal level, was shy and diffident. He was tongue-tied on formal occasions and had no small talk to ease his awkwardness with strangers. He took refuge in the telling of jokes, often funny and sometimes bawdy. He had a large collection of jokes, some for use on social occasions, others to have fun at home with his family. Connie protested when they became lewd, but Alan told them anyway.

Connie's good-natured banter defused many of Alan's furious explosions. His quick temper would evaporate if she could make him laugh. When he came home tired she would tell him all the funny things that had happened that day or repeat some joke she had heard. Her breezy impertinence was just what was needed to humour him.

From all reports it was a good marriage. Each knew how to play the game to avoid serious friction. They led separate and absorbing lives but where Connie would share the events in her life with Alan, he couldn't, or wouldn't share his.

> I think Dad and Mother were complex people. They protected each other and were very close. I remember one time Dad yelled at me, "Don't you EVER use that tone of voice to your mother!" and he glared over his glasses. He couldn't have had a better wife. But when I look back, life was, well, a sham. One dressed for dinner. Ye Gods! We did this during the Depression and just before the war; everybody was so damn proper. One hot summer night I was going out with Donald Robertson (D.E.'s son). I had bare legs and Don reproached me: "You're not wearing stockings." "No, I have a tan." "Go back and put some on." "No, if you want to take me out, I'll go, but I'm not wearing stockings."

Donald gave in. He knew there were many other young men who would gladly have taken his place. "Our beaux were ushered into the den off the front door on Dunvegan. Dad always stayed upstairs. He let mother do all the dirty work."

Life with Mother — and sometimes, Father

Both Barbara and Nancy have pleasant memories of being allowed to accompany him on his Sunday house calls. Barbara remembers:

> I often used to go with Father. It was a special treat. He'd chatter away and I'd listen. He always wore his morning coat

— stiff collar, four in hand, the whole bit. But he never had time to go to church. He worked so darn hard. It sounds funny, particularly in this day and age, to say that he had a chauffeur, but he couldn't have managed all those house calls by himself. I remember one night he had a telephone call from London and another from Hamilton and when he got back he lay down with his shoes off and his trousers on and snatched two hours rest before he had to be back at the hospital. He was great and I just adored him. We didn't get to see him much. He would be called out or he'd come in late for dinner. Norah would ask "When will the doctor will be home?" Mother would sigh, "Norah, just put it in the oven." He'd come home at hellish hours and, of course, had to eat alone and then he'd make more calls after dinner.

Dad used to take me [Nancy] with him when he made his house calls on Sunday and I was proud that I could sit alone in the car while he went in with his black bag to houses all over Toronto — nice areas, poor areas. That was a thrill for me when I was six or seven before I went to boarding school. I have some good memories like that but I did not feel comfortable with my parents. When I was a teenager and longed for advice and to feel close to them, my father was never there or he was reading medical journals in his study and I felt I wasn't important enough to disturb him. I always longed for a close family — you know, so you could go to your mother and say, "Hey, what should I do about this or that?" When you're in your teens and you have problems, that's when you need them. Once I went to mother for advice but she said, "Oh, I haven't got time for that." So I learned to solve things for myself and to keep to myself. But she was very religious. Whether it was genuine or not I don't know, but I assume it was. She said her prayers every night. The piano was on the third floor. She'd come up and play hymns when she felt like it. And I always had to go to church. We'd sit next to Dr. Starr's wife in those horrible pews at Timothy Eaton.[5]

Dad loved sports. I went to football games at Varsity Stadium with him because no one else seemed to be interested and I remember how proud he was when one year at Hatfield I won about six cups for sports. He thought that was great. I loved him dearly but I didn't really know him; I was never alone with him and I was hardly ever at home. When I wasn't at boarding school I was sent off to camp and then the war came and he wanted me to join the Navy.

Nancy seemed to be forever at cross-purposes with her parents. They were uneasy and wary in her company. Connie found it less of a strain to take Nancy to the symphony where they had little opportunity to talk.

On the other hand Connie felt totally at ease with Barbara. They were on the same wave-length. Babbling incessantly without drawing breath they chatted together, often simultaneously, but somehow neither seemed to miss a word of what the other was saying. Barbara had the easy, close relationship with her parents that her sister longed for. Nancy dared not reach out to them for fear of being snubbed. They intimidated her and seemed not to realize she wanted to be closer to them. Barbara had no such fears or inhibitions. She disarmed her parents with the spontaneous affection she was able to show.

A medical colleague, who knew the family quite well, "got the impression — and I don't remember how — that Connie was not as close to the adopted daughter as she was to her own. This unconscious partiality showed itself." Unlike the exasperation she seems to have felt towards Nancy, she had all the time in the world for Barbara who had no hesitation about asking for advice about anything and everything.

Nancy was really out of step with all of them — father, mother and sister:

Barbara and I were like oil and water. I don't know why I was always the outsider. I honestly felt I was. It just wasn't a close family but I think Mother was the best wife in the world for him. Even though they went their own ways, my parents were very close. She was very protective of him, but their interests were quite different. She went to the ballet and he read his medical journals.

Connie was an unconventional and amusing hostess, able to make her guests and even her husband relax. But at home in the city he could never forget his professional importance as completely as he was able to do at the cottage. "They used to have wonderful dinner parties. I remember them as I was flying out the front door with a date." They were splendid affairs. "He was a generous and affable host, complemented by Connie's good taste, wonderful menus and table arrangements."

Barbara was sometimes present on these splendid occasions. She remembers the time she helped her mother make an elegant decoration of fruit and flowers for the centre of the dining room table:

> One of the guests, a rich bastard — he was rude to the maids and Dad couldn't stand that — tried to pull a bunch of grapes out of the centrepiece. The whole thing toppled over and spilled across the table. Father was furious. When I asked him later, "Dad, why did you invite him?" he replied, "Because he made a big contribution to the hospital." Dad had very little interest in making money for himself but, for the hospital, he'd do anything.

The family Christmas parties were grand productions with a cast of more than thirty, including two maids from the Toronto Ladies Club in addition to Annie and Norah. The extravaganza alternated between the Browns' and the Fishers' house, Connie and Tot Fisher taking turns. Grant Fisher and a Hobbs uncle carved the turkeys, one at each end of the table. "Father couldn't carve." Mother used to say, "Oh, Alan! You never could have been a surgeon." At home Connie did all the carving because, as she said, "Your father just attacks it." None of his family seemed to realize he was faking it, that he just didn't choose to suffer the boredom of filling all those plates. Carving wood, making tables and chairs for the cabin, or filleting fish alone in his boathouse held far more appeal for his skillful hands.

Connie tried to avoid anything to do with food except at Christmas and at her special dinner parties. On these occasions her talents shone. Nothing was too much trouble. She let her imagination run rampant, obeying its commands until her energy flagged and she called a halt to further fantasies. Her enthusiasm kindled excitement and expectation in the household. At Christmastime, strings of tiny lights were draped on the trees outside and in the living room on the huge aromatic pine tree. Beneath it the presents were heaped in gaudy disarray. Two lovely old candelabra shone down on the Christmas crèche lighting the Christ child within. Candles glowed on the long dining room table set with silver, crystal and heirloom Crown Derby. There was carol singing around the piano and after the turkey dinner the families played charades.

> We'd all make asses of ourselves, but Auntie Conn didn't play. She'd be in the dining room putting away the silver and all the Christmas clutter. Finally she'd come into the living room with a triumphant smile on her face that said, "Well, I've done it and it's not my turn next Christmas."

One year when it was her turn to hold the family gathering she unintentionally escaped the responsibility. With Tot and Elisabeth she had gone over to Buffalo to buy Christmas presents and clothes. She became very ill and was in a lot of pain. A doctor came but he was unable to help her. Finally, she telephoned her husband who told her to pack her bag while he set out promptly to join her. On returning to Toronto, Alan had D.E. Robertson examine her. He made the diagnosis of bowel obstruction. Operation was immediately undertaken and the obstruction was relieved. That year, Connie spent Christmas in the hospital.

On the nineteenth of September 1942, Barbara was married to Bill Kelley at Deer Park United Church before more than a hundred and fifty wedding guests. The reception was held in the garden of the Browns' Dunvegan house. Ted Morgan, whose capacity for alcohol was unpredictable, had been asked to give the toast to the bride. His speech was amusing and appropriate until

> he stunned me by saying, "Now, you know, Alan has another beautiful daughter but she's not his." There was a shocked silence. Dad didn't do anything but the anguished expression on his face as he looked over at me said it all. I was going with Steve Gooderham at the time and I can remember how understanding he was as he put his arm around me and said, "Pay no attention." Mother was livid, her jaw clenched and I felt I could have sunk right through the grass. It was unbelievable, a real shocker.

At that moment the twenty-year friendship between the Browns and

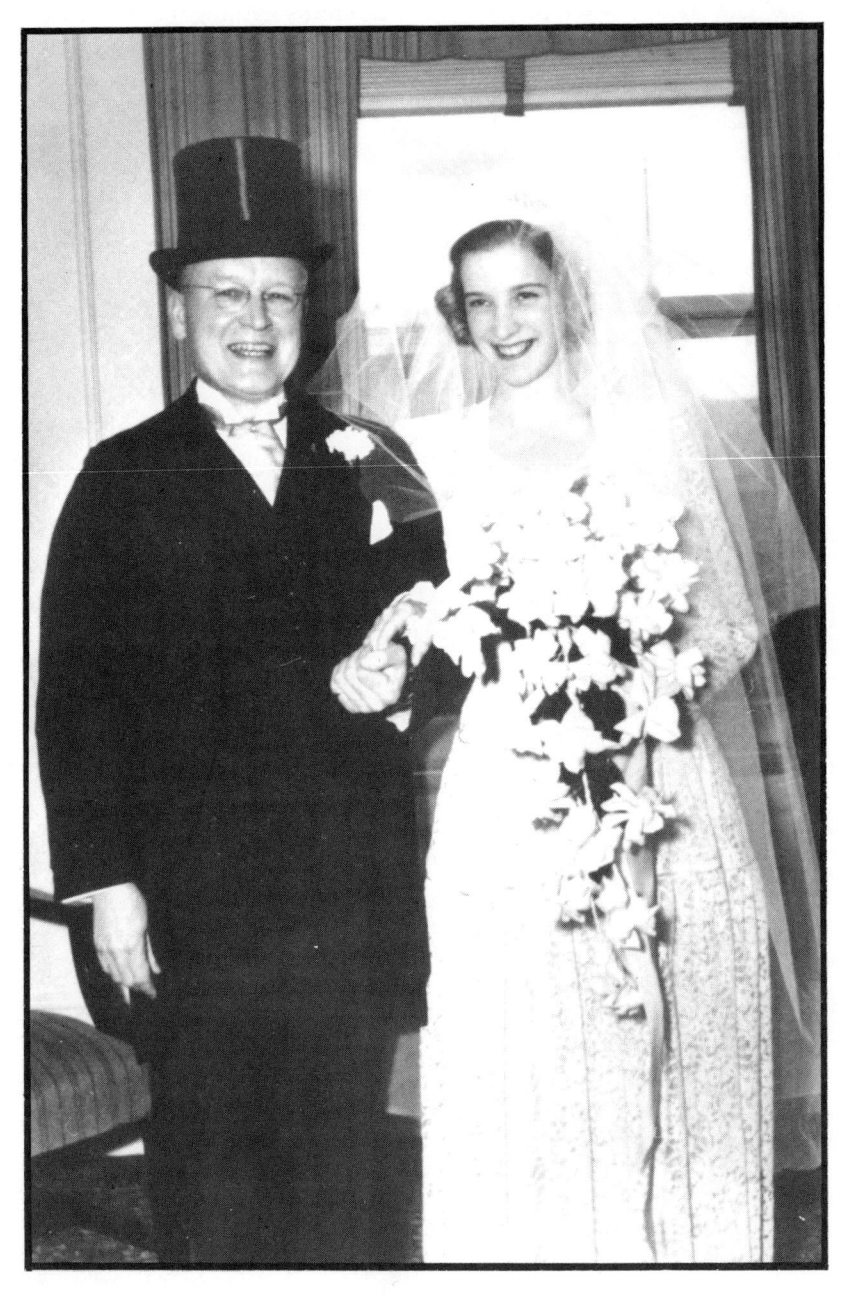

Alan with daughter Nancy on her wedding day, Vancouver, April 1944

the Morgans was broken forever. "I don't think mother ever really liked Teddy Morgan much, but she loved Aunt Gracie."[6]

In September 1941, just before Nancy joined the Navy, she was waiting for her father to come home to lunch so that he would not have to eat alone:

> I can remember that day clearly. Annie, the cook whom I adored, told me that Dad's mother had just died. Wanting to get it over with as we sat there together eating, I just blurted out, "I'm sorry, I have something awful to tell you. Your mother died this morning." He didn't seem upset. He looked at me over his glasses. "Oh?" and went on with his lunch.

Excerpt from Miss Haldenby's diary:

> Sept. 3, 1941 — Dr. B. — alone to his mother's funeral.

In 1944, while in the Navy stationed in Vancouver, Nancy married Jack Dampsey, a Naval officer. When Alan Brown had received her letter telling him about their engagement he was not pleased. His chief resident was with him in his office when he read the news. He quickly turned to his secretary, Mary Cassidy, and barked, "Find out all you can about this Dampsey fellow." Then he mumbled, "She must really love him to go through life as Nancy Dampsey!" His reaction hid the affection he could not show.

The wedding took place one spring evening in April 1944 in Vancouver and there were many guests including family and friends from the East. Nancy had tossed her Wren[7] uniform aside to appear in a traditional white gown and Barbara was a bridesmaid. As at Barbara's wedding, Dr. Brown dressed formally in tails and top hat.

Upon their return to Toronto, Alan Brown reluctantly decided that he must find less demanding work for Annie, their loyal servant and friend for more than twenty years. She was no longer the young woman who had reigned unchallenged in the kitchen and had carried out her other duties zipping about the house from basement to attic. With her incipient heart failure the house had become too big for her flagging energy. As soon as Alan and Connie had agreed on the best course for her, he went to the kitchen and gently said, "Annie, we're going to miss you very much but Mr. and Mrs Jones have fewer rooms to look after and no stairs. They would like you to work for them."

In those days there were no government pension plans. Only the rare employer could afford and chose to contribute to a private plan for their household servants. Several years earlier Dr. Brown had bought Annie an annuity but he knew she would need more income than he had been able to provide.

― Chapter 8 ―

A Falling Star

By 1950 Alan Brown was approaching the end of his long medical career as Physician-in-Chief to The Hospital for Sick Children and Professor of Paediatrics at the University of Toronto. He seemed older than his sixty-three years. In addition to fatigue from many years of crowded days, he suffered from radiation burns caused by constant use of his office fluoroscope without adequate protection. They were the days before lead shielding was taken seriously so that his finger tips began to crumble even before he retired as Chief. Many years earlier he had admitted, "If anything ever happens to my hands, I've had it." Alan Brown's fluoroscope had, little by little, destroyed the sensitivity of his finger tips and reduced his clinical skills. Nevertheless, he was still very much in control of the old hospital that he had known for forty-seven years as medical student, intern, junior staff member and finally as chief of medicine. Since the early twenties he had been gradually opening up specialty departments to encompass each new medical advance. Even so, before World War II the majority of graduating medical students had gone out into the community as general practitioners rather than as specialists. A sense of urgency to find effective treatments for the wounded during the war led to significant medical discoveries: Alexander Fleming's discovery of penicillin and its later clinical application and industrial production; new techniques in surgical treatment and mass blood transfusion; greater emphasis on dietary factors and an understanding of the

SEQUOIA
MAGNETAWAN
ONTARIO

July 12/50

Dear Michael,

Your letter was forwarded to me here — so that I can not reply on dept. note paper but I hope the end will recur its purpose — so I have not my records here you might file in the number of years when I leave the R.P.O's.

Anything else I can do for you please let me know. With kind regards

Alan Brown

SEQUOIA
MAGNETAWAN
ONTARIO

July 12/50'

To whom it may concern

Dr Lillian Sugarman Clark served on my intern staff for 2 years and I have great pleasure in stating that she was one of the best interns I have had in thirty-seven years —

(She wanted) be an asset to any pediatric staff in every respect

Alan Brown
Phys-in-Chief-*hospital*
for *Sick Ch*.

Alan's note on Connie's blue paper to Dr. Lillian Sugarman Clark with recommendation letter enclosed, July 1950

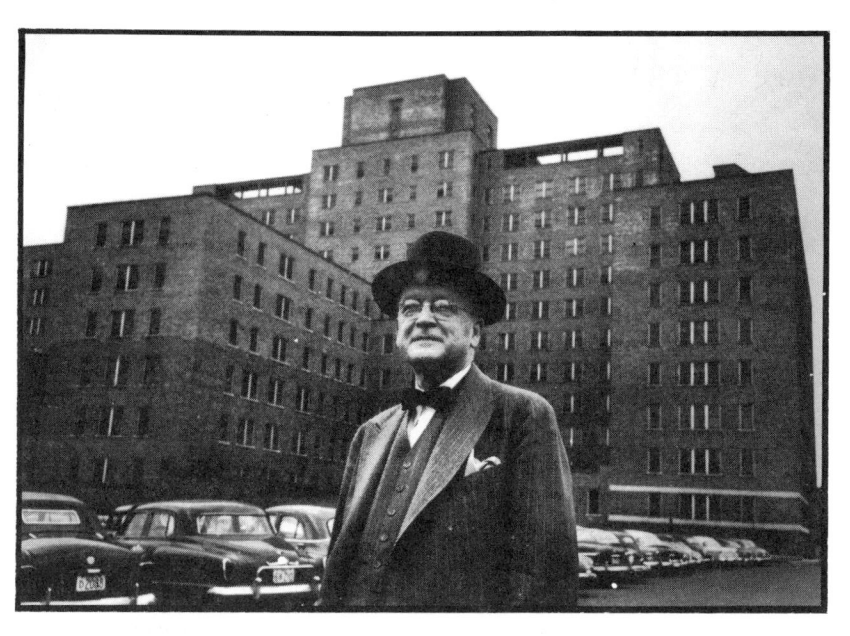

*Dream realized: Alan Brown in front of "his" new hospital
(photo H.W. Tetlow, courtesy* Maclean's Magazine*)*

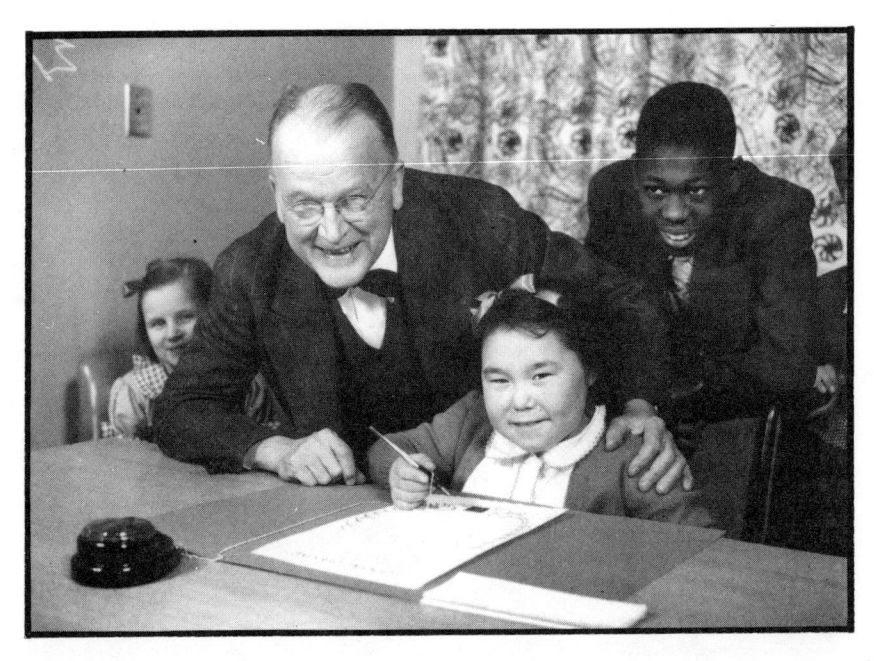

Dr. Alan Brown with three of the six patients chosen for the official opening of the new hospital on University Avenue, Globe and Mail, *16 January 1951 (Courtesy Toronto Archives)*

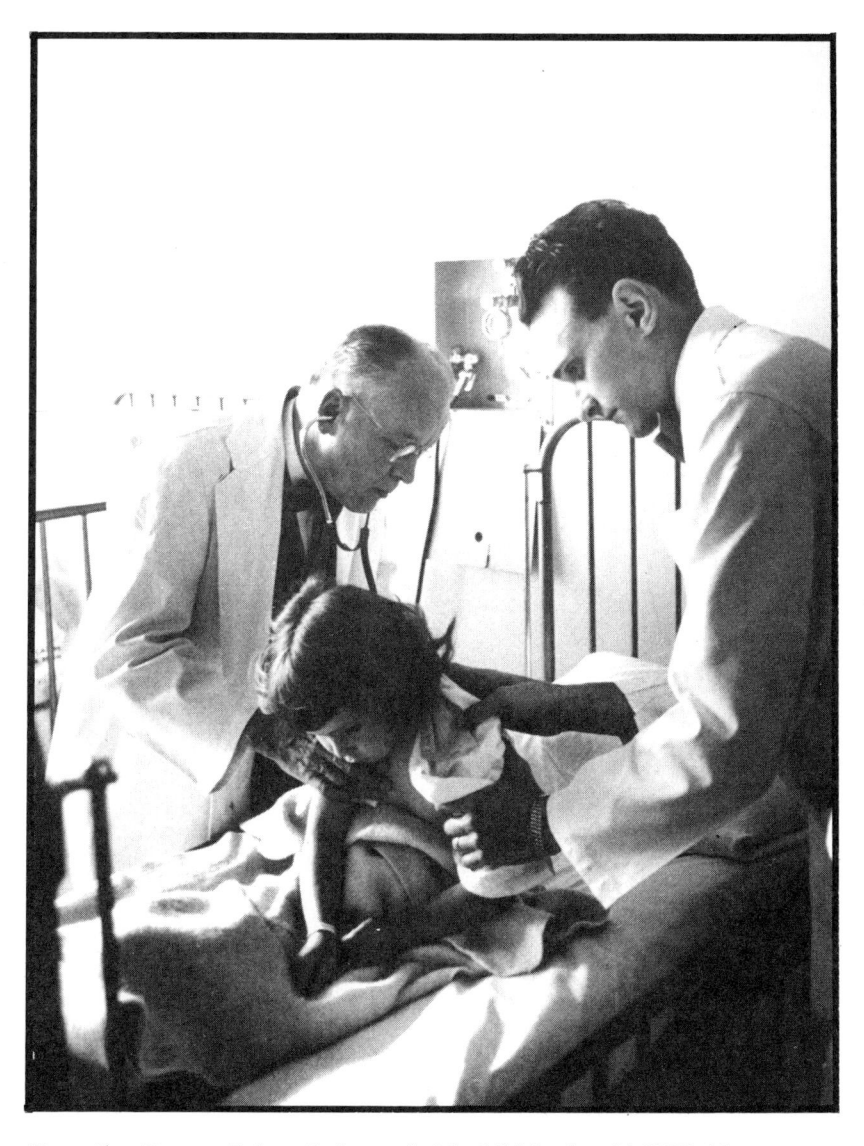

Drs. Alan Brown, Robert Farber and sick child in the old HSC (photo H.W. Tetlow, courtesy Maclean's Magazine)

psychology of stress; and techniques for the containment of epidemics. Returning veterans and other postwar students entered medicine in increasing numbers and many began to train as specialists working in the expanding departments in the old building on College Street. It was bulging at the seams trying to cater to them all.

Relief was on the way. A new hospital on University Avenue was almost ready to accept patients. Nineteen-fifty was the last year Sick Kids' operated in the College Street building, the latest in hospital design when John Ross Robertson had opened its doors in 1892. By 1917, only a quarter of a century later, it was obsolete. Throughout his long reign he had been pleading and pushing to replace the tired, run-down building — more than thirty years was a long time for this impatient man to be forced to wait. Depressions and wars had delayed its replacement, frustrating his constant efforts for renewal. In 1951 his long struggle was rewarded. At last he had his large, modern hospital. Since the 1890s the HSC had been renowned for its advanced surgical techniques. Under Alan Brown's leadership it became even more widely respected for the excellence of its paediatric medicine.

Dream Fulfilled

By 8:00 a.m. on Sunday, 4 February 1951, all was in readiness to move 193 patients from the old red stone building on College Street to the new Sick Kids' hospital on University Avenue. A light snow was falling. A camera crew from Toronto's only television station (CFTO) was impatient to film the historic event. Private cars and ambulances were poised, motors idling as they waited on Elizabeth and along Gerrard streets. In turn, they moved slowly to the side door of the old hospital. Out came the children one by one — babies in incubators, youngsters strapped on stretchers, several under oxygen tents and others in wheelchairs or hobbling along on crutches. Dr. Alan Brown, the catalyst for this strange parade, was in his element. Directing and advising he moved swiftly about in the orderly confusion until he saw the last patient carried off to the new hospital. The skillfully executed operation was completed in just two and a half hours. At 11:30 a.m. the children were being served hot Sunday dinners prepared in the new kitchens.

The dream that Alan Brown had so resolutely pursued for so many years had finally come true — but for him it was too late. He would never know every nook and cranny of the new building as he had in the old.

He worked in it only eight months. On the fourth of October 1951 he submitted his letter of resignation addressed to his old friend, Bobby Laidlaw, Chairman of the hospital's Board of Trustees:

> I wish to take this opportunity to tender my resignation as physician in chief to the hospital to become effective November 1st 1951.

The chief physician of Sick Kids' was ending his tight rule over the famous hospital. The stresses of the previous thirty-six years were collecting their dues. He was tired. From time to time he had suffered mild strokes. "He'd be away for a few days and when he returned he didn't say it was a stroke. He was too scientific for that."[1] Connie was aware of his condition and at the annual softball game between the staff and the interns "when he was up to bat his chief resident had to run for him or Mrs. Brown would yell in rebuke, 'Alan!' right in the middle of the game."[2]

Failing Health

These mild strokes had not affected his self-confidence or his control as Chief in the old building he knew so well. But in the new, he became disoriented and often had difficulty finding his way around. He was overwhelmed by its complexity and size. It was too unwieldy for his declining mental and physical energy. "The new hospital upset him. He wasn't used to it and he found it hard to change his ways."[3] His working day, which had often run to eighteen or twenty hours, shrank to eight. When he allowed it to stretch beyond this he knew his judgement was at risk. He realized he could no longer hold his expanding Department of Medicine in the palm of his hand. He was aware that he did not think as clearly and effectively as before. He was still the Physician-in-Chief and the Professor of Paediatrics but he knew that the inspiration and enthusiasm he had injected into his leadership and teaching were gone.

> One day, before he gave up, he came into my office and sat down with his head in his hands. He was completely lost and he broke down. "I just can't do it — I can't carry on." That's all he said. Seeing his distress I tried to cheer him up but he seemed to be overwhelmed.[4]

> Dear Mr Laidlaw
>
> I wish to take this opportunity to tender my resignation as Physician-in-Chief to the hospital to become effective November 1st, 1951
>
> Sincerely yours,
> Alan Brown

The end of his long reign, 1951

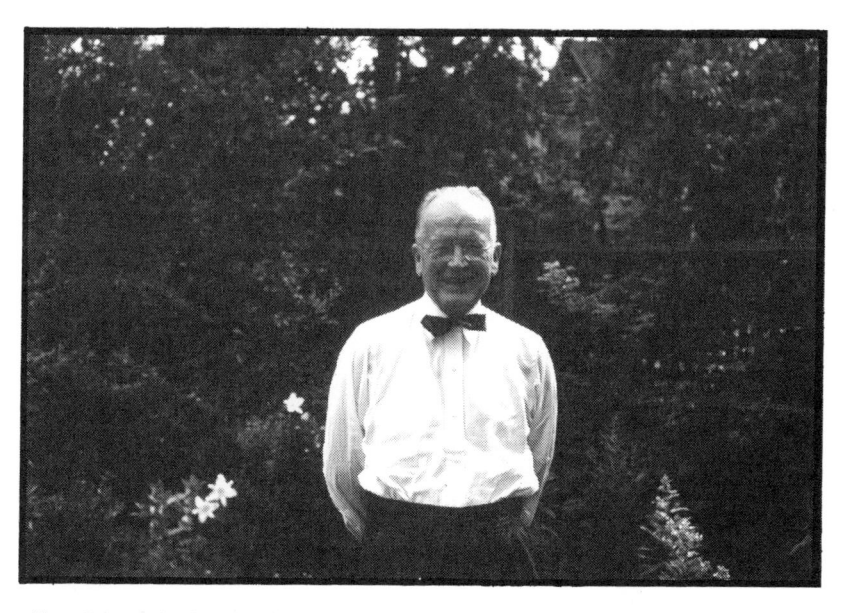

Alan Brown in his garden at 51 Dunvegan Road, Toronto (Photo: Nelles Silverthorne)

Discouraged and frightened by his deteriorating powers, his confidence crumbled. He knew many of his staff disliked him, that many wanted him to retire because his resistance to change was preventing them from prescribing new treatments and techniques. As long as Brown was in harness the hospital was marking time, unable to advance. Its energy was waning with its Chief. It was an unhappy time for Dr. Brown; he was a broken-hearted man. On his last day, white lab coat flying, he rushed out of a staff meeting in the new lecture theatre just after Nina Drake had walked by. He did not notice her as he laid his hands on the window sill to rest, looking out onto University Avenue and muttering to himself, "They'll be glad when I've gone." Mrs. Drake could not bring herself to like the man who had so unfairly treated Theo, her husband, but at that moment her heart was touched by his distress.

No Farewell for Alan Brown
A senior resident, Dr. Justin O'Brien, recalls the end ruefully. "He retired abruptly and there was no party for him, nothing at all. I don't know why. But he had rubbed a lot of people the wrong way." Phyllis Norton was indignant about the way his resignation was treated: "After all those years why didn't they give him something? Any nurse who left was given a party — even in those days!" Some interns and medical staff even refused to contribute to the cost of his portrait. He had so alienated his colleagues and bullied his staff that no one seemed to regret his departure. Surely the man who put paediatrics on the map in this country deserved to be given some kind of graceful farewell before he departed? Why was there no party and no presentation — neither a silver salver nor even a handsome humidor for his cigars? But at least there had been the face-saving coincidence of the portrait formally presented to him before anyone knew he was about to resign.

Sometime in the spring of 1951 he was asked to sit for Cleeve Horne who had been commissioned to paint the Physician-in-Chief's portrait for the Annual Meeting of The Hospital for Sick Children Alumni on the nineteenth of October.* Those in charge of the agenda thought the Alumni's first meeting in the new hospital would be an appropriate occasion to recognize Alan Brown's leadership which had led at last to the construction of the University Avenue hospital. They had no idea that

---

* In 1994 the portrait was still half hidden behind the library stacks.

he planned to offer his resignation to the Board of Trustees just two weeks before the meeting. Sir James Spence was the keynote speaker at the opening session at which Dr. Nelles Silverthorne formally outlined Dr. Brown's many achievements and presented the portrait to him before an audience made up of HSC staff and alumni, Mrs. Brown and other members of his family. His impending resignation, to take effect on the first of November, was not public knowledge on that occasion; there was no mention of it in Dr. Silverthorne's address.[5]

Thirteen days after the Annual Meeting, Alan Brown's resignation was accepted. He stepped down and Dr. A. Lawrence Chute succeeded him as Physician-in-Chief of The Hospital for Sick Children and the Professor of Paediatrics at the University of Toronto. Throughout October, his last days at the helm, Alan Brown carried on as usual in class and clinic. For some time now, in order to save his declining energy for his patients and students, he had delegated much of the administration of the hospital to its Superintendent, Joe Bower, and the supervision of the Department of Medicine to Dr. Harry Ebbs, the sole full-time staff member at that time. He had also arranged for junior colleagues to take his house and night calls. He trimmed his activities to save his energy for the day's essential demands.

On the twenty-sixth of October 1951 Alan Brown attended his last HSC Medical Advisory Board Meeting. He resigned as its chairman and announced that he would retire as Physician-in- Chief of the hospital on the 31st, five days later. He then moved the following resolution (seconded by Dr. Wansbrough) "that Dr. A.L. Chute be appointed Physician-in-Chief to The Hospital for Sick Children."

Departure

One of his senior residents, Bob Farber, vividly remembers Alan Brown's last day in front of his class:

> He was in the middle of the lecture we had prepared for him when there was a knock on the door. He was called out and presumably was told that his resignation had been accepted. We did not know this then. Since it was not uncommon for him to be summoned from a lecture to see a patient seriously ill, we just carried on. But he didn't return to his class and he never taught again. That's how it happened. The next day Dr. Chute was there.

His senior residents, Farber and Johnson, who had prepared his last lecture, were, with most of the hospital staff, stunned by his sudden departure. In some quarters, however, it was not entirely unexpected. There had been rumours flying around that he was not well. The nurse in charge of the ear, nose and throat operating room had "heard he was ill, but I just accepted his resignation as natural — he seemed like an old man to me." Three months after he had resigned as Chief he was not recognized in the hospital. "I was teaching on the fourth floor," Bernard Laski recalls, "when a man in a white lab coat walked slowly down the hall towards us. One of my students asked, 'Who's that?'." On another occasion when Alan Brown arrived to see one of his private patients, a nurse asked him who he was. His temper blew sky high and she was left shivering in her shoes.

Even before he resigned his position at Sick Kids', Alan Brown knew that it was no longer possible for any doctor to keep up with all the latest advances in paediatrics. After a time he abandoned the struggle in frustration and, eventually, in despair. A new world of paediatrics had grown up around him and so much new knowledge overwhelmed him. He no longer retired to his den to read the current medical journals before he went to bed as he had done every night of his long professional life. He knew his role as leader in the field had slowly slipped away. Younger men, often his former students, had taken the lead. Nevertheless, he retained his interest in the hospital. When Laurie Chute was head of paediatrics, "Alan would have us up to the house for dinner several times a year. Afterwards the two of us would go off to his study and he'd quiz me. He just had to know all the goings on at the hospital."

Loneliness

The last nine years of his life were increasingly sad, lonely and, near the end, distressing. From the moment he left the hospital he was a changed man. He lost his drive; it was all gone. Where he had been vibrant, positive, demanding, he now became unsure, apprehensive, even indifferent. "He just shrivelled up like a pricked balloon." His large private practice began to dwindle as new parents took their babies to the younger colleagues he had taught. Too late he realized that his loneliness in retirement was his own fault, the result of his impatient arrogance at the hospital and patronizing criticism of the paediatricians who were his rivals:

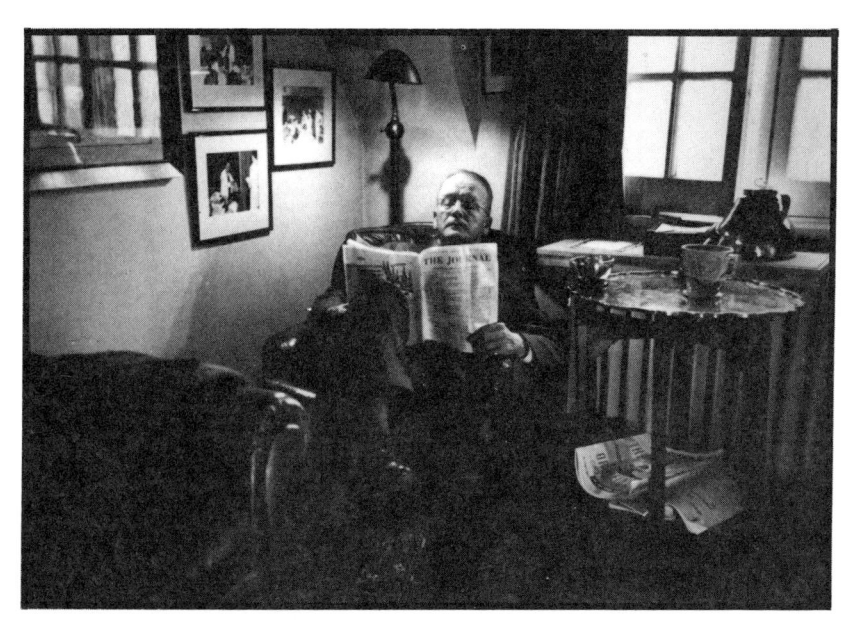

Alan Brown in his study on Dunvegan Road (photo H.W. Tetlow, courtesy Maclean's Magazine)

> He had antagonized so many of us that he really was a very lonely man. Over the years Alan and I had often tangled but I went up to see him several times after he retired and he was so happy to see me that I'm sure he was lonely.[6]

One of the Sick Kids' research staff was bitter: "He didn't do anything to make himself loved." Not many of his former associates continued any kind of contact with him. He received fewer and fewer of their referrals. "He had no friends when he retired — none — because he'd goosed so many of his colleagues."

Not even those who really liked him took the time to visit. Nelles Silverthorne regrets his neglect. He does not know why he did not go up to see him more than once or twice. Ted Morgan, then living out of town, may have gone occasionally but their friendship had been severely strained by Morgan's unseemly speech at Barbara Alan Brown's wedding in 1942. The only other paediatricians Alan saw socially were younger colleagues and former students, particularly Laski, O'Brien, Weinberg and Farber, all of whom, during the fifties, had assisted him with his private practice by taking his house calls and, in the summer, attending to his office. Gus O'Brien visited him a couple of times. He had accompanied him on three out-of-town consultations when he was still the Chief. "He did all the driving — I was fascinated by tales of his postgraduate years in New York and Germany. He was a different Dr. Alan Brown in his mellow, twilight years." Bob Farber was invited over for a drink at least twice when Alan Brown was at home alone.

> It was Christmas Eve. I remember he was wearing his smoking jacket when he answered the door. We sat in his den with a drink and he was very upset as he reminisced about things that had happened years before. We talked about some of his staff who didn't like him, about Manace being fired for good reasons but who bitterly criticized him to any staff member who would listen. He regretted the long wait Jack Slavens endured before he received an appointment; "At least Jack knows it really wasn't my fault." He was depressed that he had been so little liked, that his former staff spoke so disparagingly of him.

Connie, accustomed to travelling or to spending her days and evenings without him, didn't let his retirement interfere with her life. When she was not travelling she was occupied with her many charitable and social activities. However, in the late afternoons when he returned from his office in the Medical Arts Building, she was nearly always at home and ready as usual to distract and amuse him with the events of her day while they relaxed with a glass of sherry before being called in to dinner. Afterwards, she went to the theatre or the symphony as she had always done, but not with Alan. To change her way of life so that she could be at home more often did not occur to her, while he would not admit that he was lonely when she went out in the evening or when she was trotting around antique shops in Europe. In fact he encouraged her to lead the life she had always led.

Depression and Drinking
When Connie was away, often his only friend to share the evenings was a bottle of sherry that he finished off while reading in bed. Formerly he had drunk sparingly but soon after retiring he had it delivered by the case. When Connie was at home the sherry took second place and he contentedly spent the evening with her or with other family members. Occasionally they entertained their non-medical friends such as the Bakers, the Laidlaws or the Woods. Gordon Gallie, an obstetrician, had been a close friend ever since 1909 when they interned together at Sick Kids'. Later, when Connie and Marion Gallie became friends, the Gallies were uncle and aunt to Barbara and Nancy. After Alan Brown resigned as Physician-in-Chief the two couples continued their long friendship until two years before Alan died when something happened to cool it permanently. The reason soon became clear.

Slowing Down
His domestic life in some disarray, his private practice sliding into dull routine and his health failing, Alan increasingly depended on his junior colleagues to carry out his treatment instructions and to keep him informed about the progress of his patients.

> When I started to practise in July of 1950, he asked me if I would make his house calls for him. He took the summer off and I ran his office. He asked me if I'd like to have an office there but I refused. Jews were not wanted in the Medical Arts and I didn't

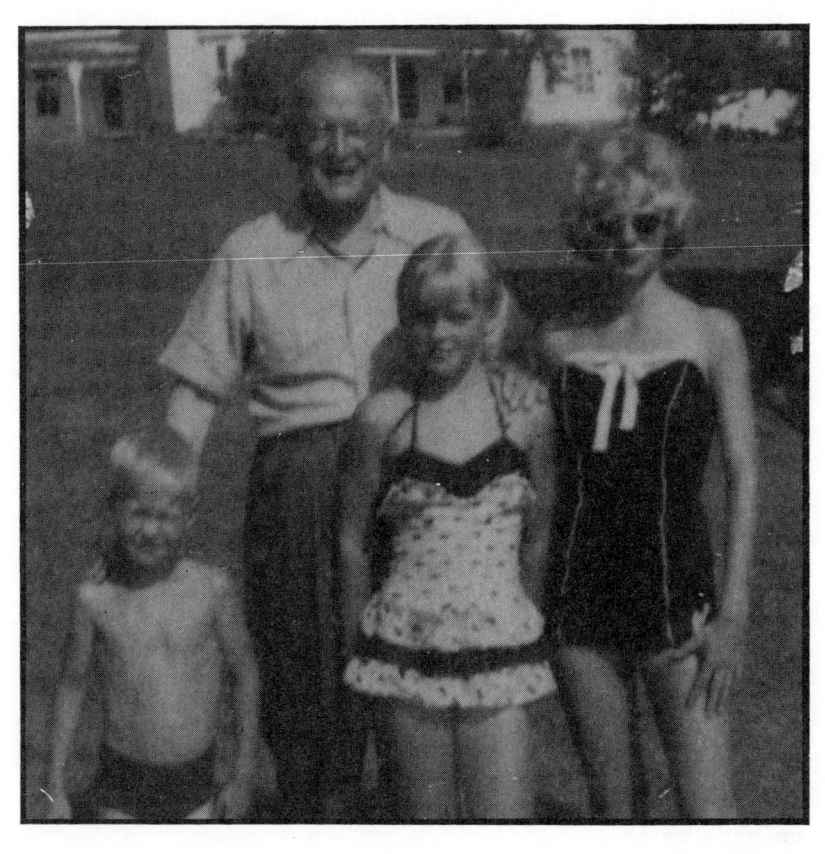

Alan Brown with grandchildren Tim, Stephanie and Ann Kelley about 1957

want any special privileges. One day in the early fifties I was on Major Street making a house call. I checked back with my answering service and found there was a message from Alan Brown. I called him at home and in a solemn voice he said, "I looked up Joy's medical record." Long pause. "She has no allergies. Marry her." He gave a short toast at our wedding and once came for dinner when Mrs Brown was out of town. After he died she telephoned to say he'd left me a couple of books. One was the biography of Abraham Jacobi, the grand old man of American paediatrics.[7]

Now that her father was no longer fully occupied with patients, Barbara was happy to have him spend more time with her family. She and her husband Bill "often had my parents for dinner and our three kids used to wrestle with him. They adored him. Tim wanted to get old enough to smoke a cigar with Gramps." As his practice decreased he frequently dropped by to see her in the afternoons. "We'd sit in the kitchen drinking coffee and I'd tell him all the silly things the children had done since we'd last seen him."

A Bittersweet Conclusion

Alan Brown had no interests outside the hospital and his profession, except his beloved cabin on Ahmic Lake. Now that he could spend more time there he found all the problems of maintaining the rambling log cabin were no longer interesting challenges but unwelcome burdens. He and Connie wanted Barbara or Nancy to take it over but neither was able to do so. After a prostatectomy in the spring of 1953 he quietly savoured his last summer along the Magnetawan. In late August he and Connie drove over to a cottage where Barbara and her husband were visiting friends. "Dad was smiling and seemed pleased when he told us they'd sold the cabin to a fraternity brother from Baltimore."

No more fishing, canoeing, sailing through the lazy summer days on Ahmic Lake or along the Magnetawan. He had no hobbies other than making furniture for the cabin. Gone was the careless freedom of the casual life at the cottage. He would miss his medical friends summering around Magnetawan and the friendships he had built among the local inhabitants, the Raaflaubs and George White, his handy man. A few weeks at Elgin House or The Briars in summer, Sea Island, Georgia or

Florida in winter would not be satisfying substitutes.

He had always dreamed of writing a book on the effects of weather on the behaviour of children. It was to be based on the research in several papers that he and Fred Tisdall had given twenty years earlier. The plan was still-born. Now that he had the time it was too late. The self-discipline that he had always been able to muster was failing with his energy.

Family Problems and Pleasures
He was aware that his daughters had problems but they were not of the medical kind he was accustomed to solving. He felt inadequate, not knowing how to respond to their personal difficulties. Nancy relates:

> We were up at the cottage when I was getting a divorce. Now that was one time when he did sit down and we talked. In my misery I wasn't so scared of him, I guess. At the end he spoke, "Well, I knew a long time ago that you and Jack weren't getting on, that there was something wrong," and I burst out, "Well, why didn't you say so? I thought I was going mental." He said, gently, "Because, Tiny, I knew you could cope." And that's why I always felt I must never let him down.

A more distressing memory of her parents lingers with Nancy. She was up at Sequoia with her two little girls, three and one:

> It was just after Jack and I had split up. I know Dad was upset about it and I was feeling pretty depressed myself. (Dr.) Bill Greenwood helped me. He said I wasn't going crazy. Anyway, it was about nine at night. Debby and Diana were asleep. I paddled over to the Littles, just two cottages away and had been there for an hour or so when Father came crashing through the woods and thundered up onto their verandah. He roared at me in front of my friends for not coming home. I was twenty-nine-years old and so embarrassed to be treated like a child! I paddled back and I remember him lying on the couch beside the fireplace very red in the face and mother saying, "Of course, you know you've nearly killed your father." I felt guilty but I didn't know why he was so angry. I was afraid he'd have a heart attack. I was very hurt. "I was only visiting friends; don't you

trust me?" He didn't explain and I never apologized. At that moment all I wanted was to get away from there.

This unhappy incident was one of Nancy's last memories of the cabin on Ahmic Lake. Fred Weinberg put it down to Alan's inability to come to terms with Nancy's divorce. "His daughters upset him a lot with their personal problems."

Alan Brown's grandchildren gave him a great deal of pleasure — in small doses. He sometimes allowed them to play and crawl all over him as Barbara's little Ann, Stephanie and Tim did. They have many tender memories of him. Stephanie says she loved to sniff the smoke from his cigars and Tim remembers his gentle jesting: "Are you old enough to smoke a cigar with me?" Nancy's daughters, Debby and Diana, gleefully responded to his teasing and jokes at the weekly Sunday dinners at their grandparents' house. They joined in with him when he began one of his familiar admonitions, "No cakes, candies, ice ceam, cookies. . . ." They knew the litany by heart.

Hurricane Hazel

By the mid-fifties his office nurse and receptionist, Doris and Grace Haldenby, noticed he was becoming slow, moody and difficult. He wasn't pushing himself as he used to nor was he tearing around between office and hospital, and he had others taking his house calls. A brief entry in Grace's diary comments on his declining strength:

> October 15, 1954 — Hurricane Hazel — Dr. B walked home from Med Arts and it nearly killed him.

It was the most devastating storm in Toronto's history. It claimed seventy-eight lives. Miss Haldenby's entry did not exaggerate Dr. Brown's brush with death. He had no idea what was in store for him. That morning the weather office had predicted "the intensity of this storm has decreased . . . and should no longer be classified as a hurricane . . . it will pass just east of Toronto before midnight."[8] By early evening six inches of rain had fallen and winds were gusting up to seventy miles per hour. Toronto traffic was at a standstill. It took two or three hours to travel by car from Queen to College Street, a distance of less than a kilometre. Churches and synagogues became relief shelters. Northwest of the city, below Woodbridge, a dam broke. Torrents of water swept down the Humber Valley washing away forty bridges and creating havoc in the lowlands. Lambton Golf Course looked like the Everglades. A helicopter lifted out six bodies. In Etobicoke the water boiled down Raymore Drive nearly six feet deep crashing through houses and leaving thirty-six dead.

Brown's battle to get home was a nightmare. Transformers were exploding, huge fallen trees and hydro poles dangling hot wires criss-crossed the roads along his route. The railway underpass at Dupont Street was five feet below the surface of the water. Along its raised pedestrian walkway he sloshed through puddles and assorted debris and could dimly see the tops of stranded cars in the swirling flood waters below him under the bridge. He wondered if he could make the long climb back to his house on Imperial Street still a mile away above St. Clair Avenue. After wading through the knee-deep stream flowing across the bottom of Poplar Plains Road he finally reached higher ground. Instead of his normal half hour, two hours after leaving his office he stumbled through his front door to sink exhausted on the nearest chair.

Grace Haldenby's terse description of Alan Brown's ordeal was the last entry in her diary until just before he closed his private practice four years later. He became increasingly difficult throughout those years. She explains, gently euphimistic, "He was unwell much of the time."

> There were times [Nancy remembers] when he was sick and he used to watch wrestling. I would tease him. He was death on television: "It is dreadful — kills the brain cells." But he finally bought a set when they moved to Imperial. I remember going over to see him one time when he was confined to bed. "I don't believe you're watching wrestling!" and he laughed. "I love it, it's relaxing."

By the mid-fifties most of his patients were teenagers or even young adults. One woman remembers she continued with Dr. Brown until after she was married. Robert Farber, one of his junior colleagues who took his night and house calls, watched the decline of patients he saw for him during his last years from two or three a night to two or three a month. It came to Grace Haldenby that she had not put an infant on the scales for a long time. She remembers being told that he was found one day at his desk with his hands over his face, silently weeping because he had nothing to do, no consultations or anything.

Depression Deepens

His depression was exacerbated by his frequent drinking bouts that began after his retirement from the hospital. "A lot of successful people drink when they feel themselves slipping. We've even had some doctors at Sick Kids' come into the staff room inebriated."[9] Nancy wishes she had not been so busy trying to put her own life together that she had no time to help her father:

> Mother was always away in Europe or the States with Auntie Tot or Auntie Ber. She may have realized that he needed her, that he was depressed, but she ignored it as she ignored most inconvenient things. There used to be an awful lot of cases of Paarl sherry. I think he was a troubled person really. He would phone me, bombed to the eyeballs. I used to think maybe he was lonely and I remember thinking, "Oh dear, why are you doing this?" But I had my own problems with children and job and worrying about both. All the same I wish I'd gone down to see him when he was alone like that. That might have been the time when I could have got close to him.

Remembering, Barbara plays down that unhappy time. "Before Bill and I took him up to Homewood that June he was tending to take too much."

In February, three months before he was admitted to Homewood, Alan sent Nelles Silverthorne a postcard from Florida where he and Connie were on holiday. It showed a small, hen-pecked man in the back seat of a car driven by his wife. Silver at first thought Alan was poking fun at himself but then felt the laugh was probably on him, Nelles, with his wife Betty at the wheel. In either case, he had treasured the postcard for more than thirty years, through all Alan's bursts of arrogance, temper and ingratitude, as a memento of his life-long respect and devotion to a man whose failings he recognized but whom he was always ready to defend.

Alan Brown Accepts an Old Friend's Advice

For several months his family and his few close associates worried about his increasingly frequent periods of depression. Grace admits, "He may

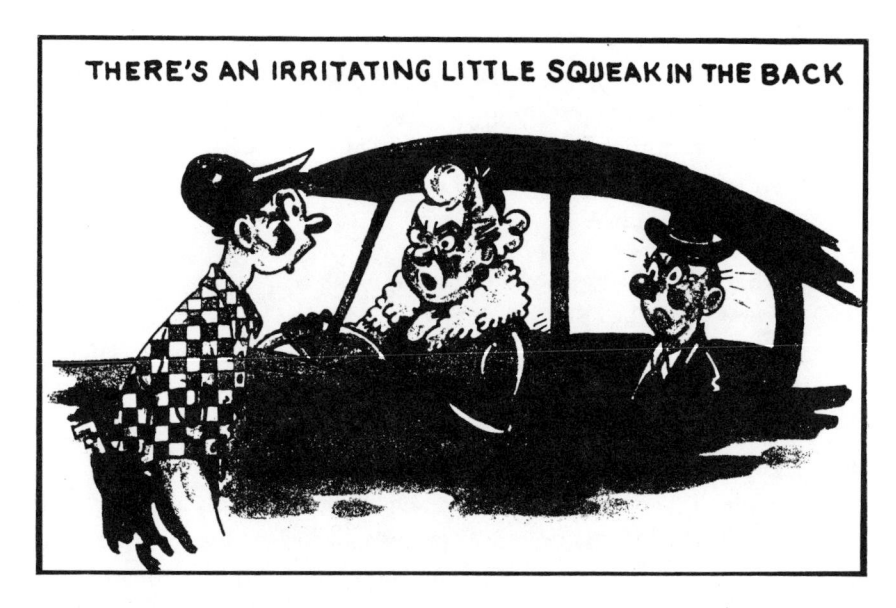

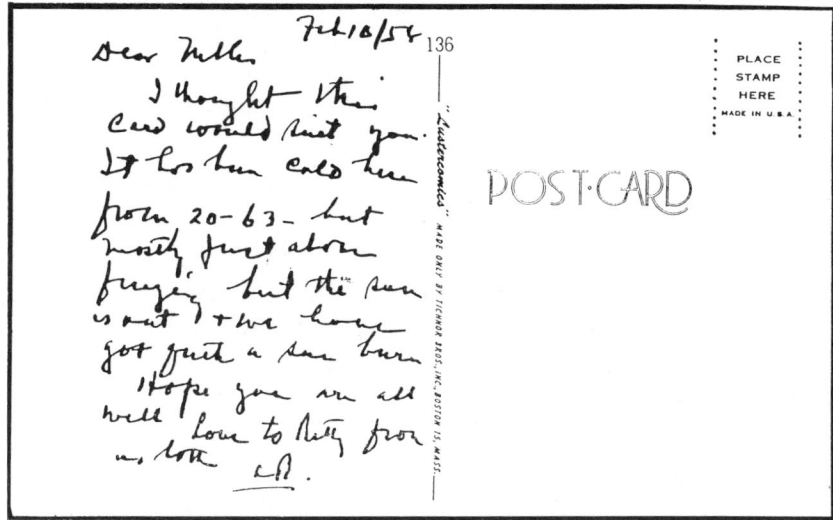

"Who is the pipsqueak?" Florida, February 1958: postcard from Alan Brown to Nelles Silverthorne

have known he wasn't quite right, that there was something wrong. There was a sort of half-way period; I mean, he didn't suddenly go nuts overnight." His old friend Gordon Gallie went for a walk with him one day and quietly suggested, "Alan, we're worried about you. Don't you think you had better go to Homewood?" Alan had great respect for Dr. Gallie and his advice was heeded, but from that moment the easy friendship between the Browns and the Gallies became only a memory. "All of a sudden Mother's feelings toward Uncle Gordon and Aunt Marion changed. The closeness was no longer there." No doubt Connie wanted to avoid them out of embarrassment — because they knew too much about Alan's problems.

Homewood

Alan Brown made the decision himself and arranged to be admitted to the Homewood Health Centre, at that time a private hospital for mental and emotional disorders, including alcoholism. He kept his decision secret until the last moment. He knew Connie would not be able to take the news without great distress. On the fifth of June 1958, Barbara and Bill drove him to Homewood. By the time he was admitted to Homewood nearly seven years had passed since he had retired from The Hospital for Sick Children, but his name was still well known in the medical community. Rumours were whispered that he was receiving shock treatment for depression and some even hinted he might have attempted suicide.

Since he was no longer in the bright light of public attention, few were aware that he had been suffering from severe depression. His family tried to keep his hospitalization and treatment secret, to hide what was all too often regarded as shameful or a deficiency of self-discipline. The day of enlightenment is still awaited.

In acute depression, even without evidence of attempted or contemplated suicide, all personal articles that could be used to harm a patient are removed by the hospital staff. No exception was made for Alan Brown. When Nancy visited him, she remembers:

> I spoke to him and felt close to him and he hugged me. He looked like a little bird, chirping to hide his embarrassment. "Tiny, isn't it awful? They won't even let me have a tie or a pair of nail scissors or anything." He said he'd had shock treatments and he kind of apologized to me, he was so embarrassed and

upset. Then I leaned over and kissed him, told him I loved him. He didn't know what to say but looked up with a smile. "That's fine, Tiny." It was such a bare room and Mother standing there all a-twit. When we got home, she said, "You must not tell anyone. No one must know what happened and no one must know he's there. I mean, what would people say?" I blew my stack, "What's there to be ashamed of? Who cares what anybody thinks! He's a great man. Can't you admire him for having the guts to say he needed help? Can't you be proud of him?" I was furious — Barbara and Mother facing me in my own living room, stressing that I must tell no one.

Perhaps Connie and Barbara were right. Alan Brown himself might have wanted to hide his condition behind a wall of secrecy. It would certainly have been in character. Throughout his professional life he had tried to cover up or ignore his mistakes. He would hardly want to reveal an infirmity, especially a disorder that finally convinced him to seek help in what many still call a mental hospital. One relative who respected his desire for privacy and his wish to keep his whereabouts secret decided not to visit him at Homewood.

At Homewood he was given two shock treatments. "He told me the staff were quite amazed that he didn't go sort of bonkers. He didn't enjoy them but said they didn't bother him much and he was right with it when he came out of there" — a faithful daughter's confident assessment offered to hide the extent of her father's emotional instability and to save the family's face. The shock treatments had helped to overcome his depression but did nothing for his increasing confusion and failing memory.

Alan Brown returned home 19 June 1958. He and Connie immediately arranged a few weeks' holiday at The Briars, a resort on the shores of Lake Simcoe, where they had rented a cottage right on the edge of the golf course. Here at last he was able to indulge in the game he had rarely had time to play. His early interest in it many years before had resulted in his contributing the Alan Brown Golf Trophy, for many years presented annually to the winning HSC staff member.

Alan Brown's Stroke
One afternoon in early September when he arrived at his office, the Hal

denby sisters observed that his walk was unsteady; he shuffled, almost staggered along and his speech was affected. This persisted for several weeks and although patients and their mothers did not seem to notice, some of the other tenants in the Medical Arts Building began to ask the Haldenbys what was wrong with Dr. Brown: perhaps he had sprained his ankle? Doris and Grace covered for him as well as they could, but it was obvious to them that he had had a stroke. While he tried to ignore the signs of a stroke they had to put up with his more frequent bursts of temper and increasing forgetfulness:

> He didn't seem to understand that he wasn't himself. I don't think he realized he was forgetful. This made it very hard for us. He was making a lot of small mistakes but he was getting very canny at that stage and able to cover them a bit. He was being awfully difficult with the patients by then and he was much more dependent. We did everything we could to help him, not hustling him and that sort of thing.

His colleagues Chute, Laski, Silverthorne and Weinberg discussing his symptoms, concluded the sporadic attacks that had kept him home for a few days over the years were small strokes. The cumulative effect of these little strokes (transient ischaemic attacks in medical jargon), added to the recent more severe attack, accounted for the disability of mind and body Grace Haldenby had described.

The Last Straw
Trying to be helpful one afternoon in the office, Grace brought Alan Brown's attention to a remark written on a patient's history:

> I think it was Dr. Silverthorne's handwriting. Anyway, it irritated him and he blew up at me. "I don't need that. I know more about medicine than Silverthorne will ever know." At this moment I thought, "To heck with it!" I don't think I ever spoke to him again. That time in my life with him was very difficult, so painful I've tried to blot it out. He always had to be right. There was a time when something he did was wrong, but he had been so positive about it, it nearly killed him when he realized he had made a mistake.

"An Odd Family"

Grace Haldenby was not surprised when she learned that neither Nancy nor Barbara had ever noticed that their father had had a mild stroke resulting in a seaman's stagger and slurred speech. Barbara later confessed that "Grace would know because she was with him all day, but I never knew and Mother never told me." And Nancy admitted she "went there for dinner with the girls nearly every Sunday and we didn't notice anything unusual."

> They are an odd family. But I suppose he could have driven home and into his garage, slipped in the back door, through the house to his study and then sat reading his journals. He was a very clever man and would know how to hide it. I don't think he would tell Mrs. Brown. She must have known but she would think it was up to him to tell Nancy and Barbara and if he didn't, she wouldn't. Besides, Doris and I would notice his condition and could keep an eye on him.

One person knew about his stroke — Nina Drake:

> When Theo was bedridden for eighteen months with all the symtoms of a stroke, Alan Brown phoned me. I was someone he never really knew and never had any time for. He was half weeping the way stroke victims do and desperate to talk to somebody. I had my hands full at home with Theo but I remember his calling. He needed someone to talk to.

Private Practice Closes

Sometime in late September of 1958 Alan Brown reluctantly faced the fact that his life as a doctor was finished. Abrupt as always, he gave no warning before announcing he was closing his office at the end of October. The Haldenbys were astounded:

> He just walked out on us one day, saying, "I'm not coming back any more. Cut off the telephones." Wouldn't you think he'd wake up the next morning and think, "My God! What are all my patients going to do?" How on earth did he think we could cope without a telephone? What absolutely infuriated me was

his indifference to his patients. They all had typed appointments given to them months, even a year in advance. Some of them had to come down by dogsled — well, not quite, but it was a big effort. We had to stop them. We worked nights but some we couldn't reach and it was awful. The other doctors were very good. They tried to see whoever they could and took over the responsibility for some of the office furniture and equipment. It was a very difficult time. I got terribly fed up with him. He really left the most awful mess.

Alan offered his remaining practice to Silverthorne who reports: "'Nelles, I want you to take over. I'm going to give you all my histories.' I replied, 'I'd like your practice but I can't take your histories. I've no place to put them all.'" Unwell though he was, Brown's usual determination did not falter. Silver took the histories, many annotated by Brown. When Silverthorne himself retired about 1985 he gave the files with his own to his associate paediatrician, Ross Johnson. Johnson recently checked his dead files boxed in his garage but did not turn up any of Alan Brown's histories. The last entry in Grace Haldenby's diary reads:

Oct. 31/58. Moving day at the office. Got the histories all filed away. Many are very personal and I worry about them.

The Last Lap
Two or three days before he died Connie and Alan were invited out to the Chutes' farm. The September evening was warm and clear and the four old friends sat on the stone terrace with their drinks before dinner. There they reminisced as they watched the sun set across the valley :

We talked about their cottage near Magnetawan and the time Laurie and I visited with them there. The following Monday or Tuesday Alan came into Laurie's office. He had brought a dozen little butter spreaders that they'd had at their cottage. He told Laurie he wanted him to have them to remember the nice times we'd had together. He had a gentle warmth that he didn't show at the hospital or in his teaching.

The end, when it came, was sudden. Barbara recounts his final hours :

> He was seventy-two or three when it happened. He'd driven up to see us on Glengrove. We talked and had a cup of coffee and he seemed absolutely fine while he was here. As he was driving away I happened to glance out the living room window. I was horrified. He drove up on the kerb, then abruptly veered back to the street. It was so unlike him. I couldn't do anything. I couldn't run after the car. He drove himself down to Imperial. I phoned mother and their maid answered: "Yes, Mrs. Kelley, your father is here. I don't think he's feeling very well. I had to help him in the door." I flew down. Mother was in a panic. He was turning bright red in the face and I went to get cold cloths. If I spoke loudly enough he could hear and he thanked me. He kept repeating, "Thank you, you're very kind," and I'd say, "Father dear, don't talk. I just want to keep you cool." I went down to the hospital with him. Mother was terrified of hospitals and stayed at home. She knew and I knew he was going to die. I looked in his room. There was a nurse with him and he was absolutely purple in the face. I dashed to the desk: "I think he's going — someone please notify my mother." Moments later Barney Barnett came out of the room with George Boddington, an anaesthetist at the General. Barney said, "Barbara, Dr. Boddington says he can keep your father alive for twenty-four hours." I replied, "Oh! my God, no! I mean — why?"

Barbara understood the need for death. She would not allow life-support systems to be applied for her father. Many years later George Boddington, remembering that fateful day, said that Alan Brown's brain was dead when he was brought in; his pupils were dilated and fixed.

Laurie Chute reflects:

> When he died they found some occlusion of his carotid arteries. If he had had reduced blood supply to his brain over a period of years and if his carotid arteries were slowly becoming blocked, this may have been one of the reasons he resigned from Sick Kids'. He felt he no longer had the mental capacity to run the show.

Honoured in Death

Alan Brown died on Wednesday, 7 September 1960, three weeks before his seventy-third birthday. The funeral service was held at Deer Park United Church. While Connie, Barbara and Nancy were being driven over to the service, Connie was weeping. It was a big funeral. The procession was led by Nelles Silverthorne followed by Alan's close friends, Eddy Baker and Bobby Laidlaw, then eight or nine medical colleagues.

The church was overflowing that bright, warm day in early September. The premier of Ontario, Leslie Frost, the mayor of Toronto, Nathan Phillips, and many other elected members of the provincial and local governments turned out to honour Dr. Alan Brown. There were officials from all the primary health care groups, many of which Alan Brown had established many years before. The staffs of The Hospital for Sick Children and the University of Toronto were fully represented. The largest group of all would have pleased Alan Brown the most — his patients. From all walks of life they came to attend the last rites of the man who in many cases had saved their lives or their children's lives.

> I remember the dwarfs, and other old patients who brought their children. I saw how many people loved him. He really was a god to so many and yet there were a great many others who just couldn't stand him.[10]

Respect and admiration continued in the eulogies of the city's newspapers as they recounted the many accomplishments of Alan Brown's long professional life. He was called the father of paediatrics in Canada by all his contemporaries. At the time of his retirement approximately seventy-five percent of the practising paediatricians in Canada had received part or all of their training under his leadership.[11] Bobby Laidlaw remembered his friend with a graceful memorial, a stained glass window[12] in the tiny HSC chapel. Discreet backlighting makes its colours glow in the dimly-lit room and its bronze plaque declaims:

TO THE GLORY OF GOD AND IN MEMORY OF
DR. ALAN BROWN PHYSICIAN-IN-CHIEF 1919 — 1951
AND HIS COLLEAGUES GIVEN BY A FRIEND

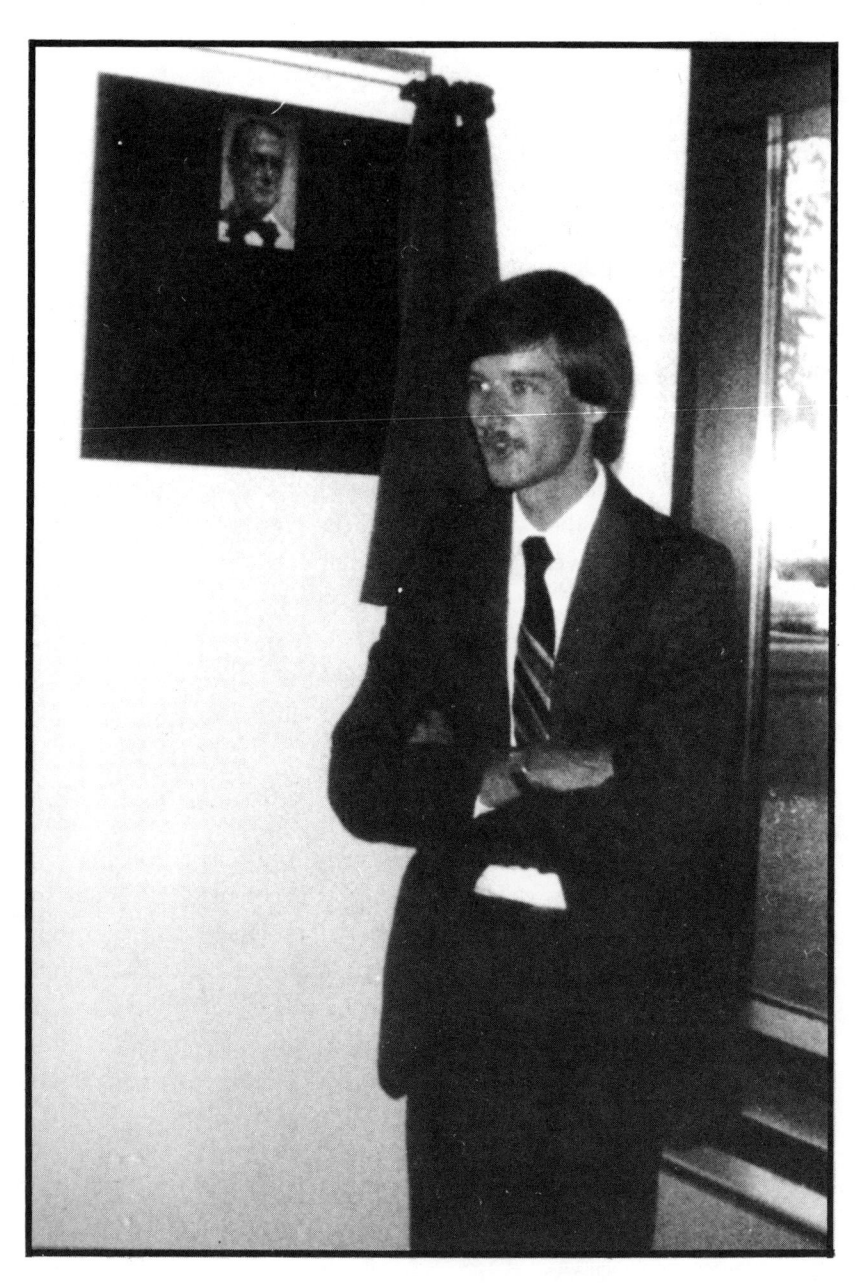

Tim Kelley unveils plaque dedicating 77 Elm Street to his grandfather

The Hospital for Sick Children designated a curious anomaly — a parking garage and a residence for medical staff — as the Alan Brown building. In its small lobby a brass plaque, unveiled by his grandson Tim Kelley, recognizes his grandfather's long reign as Physician-in-Chief. Outside the building a large sign merely publicizes "HSC PARKING" and another in large black letters reads, "77 ELM STREET".

Alan Brown's fame has not endured. Thirty-five years after his death his name is no longer the household word it once was. Medical history has treated him shabbily, his achievements now largely forgotten. Even in his beloved Hospital for Sick Children his portrait, painted by Cleeve Horne, has been tucked away in the stacks, partly hidden behind a desk in the hospital's library he helped to create.

Alan Brown is buried in Mount Pleasant Cemetery in the same plot as his close friend and brother-in-law, Grant Fisher, who had died several years earlier. Lying on the ground above his grave is a small flat stone — difficult to find and partly overgrown by grass. The weathered letters can barely be traced with a finger:

ALAN GOWANS BROWN
SEPT. 27. 1886 — SEPT. 7. 1960
BELOVED HUSBAND OF
CONSTANCE HOBBS

Connie lived for sixteen more years

> but life ended for her when Uncle Alan died. She had been crazy about him ever since she was sixteen or seventeen. Because he received no money from the hospital or the university, Uncle Alan had bought her an annuity years before and she had a little from her own family as well as his life insurance.[13]

His estate was probated at $132,000. Many unpaid fees were never settled, including some outstanding accounts owed by wealthy patients. "However, Auntie Conn had a maid so I don't think she was strapped," a niece dryly observed.

During the summer of 1991 Nancy was staying with friends on Ahmic Lake. They paddled over to visit Alan Brown's cherished cabin.

It looked exactly the same on the outside and still had Dad's handcarved "Sequoia" above the French doors on the verandah. The Leverings, who had bought it from us, were still there. They were very nice but I didn't accept their invitation to go inside. Dad's mahogany boat, the AlCon, looked as good as new but they had it up for sale.

Memories crowded into her mind, especially of the outdoor life he loved. "I could almost see him — fishing, canoeing, sailing and puttering around. I felt like crying, but I was glad I went."

Conclusion
Pioneer Forgotten

"Nobody has contributed more to children's welfare than Alan. He developed the whole field of paediatrics in Canada. There he was with everything — but because of his personality he destroyed himself in the end." *Dr. W.A. Hawke*

Dr. Alan Brown laid the foundations of paediatrics in the days when bedside skills were paramount in medical practice, and he gathered a staff whose scientific contributions gave his hospital a world-wide reputation for paediatric excellence.

His arrogant and autocratic style, originally so effective, became a liability when the rapid progress of medical science overtook him and he could no longer control the specialty he had created.

Yet the clinical and diagnostic skills which Alan Brown had mastered and strove to pass on to his students are more important than ever today. Technology cannot replace them.

In the end, his abrasive personality cost him the cachet he deserved — The Grand Old Man of Canadian Paediatrics.

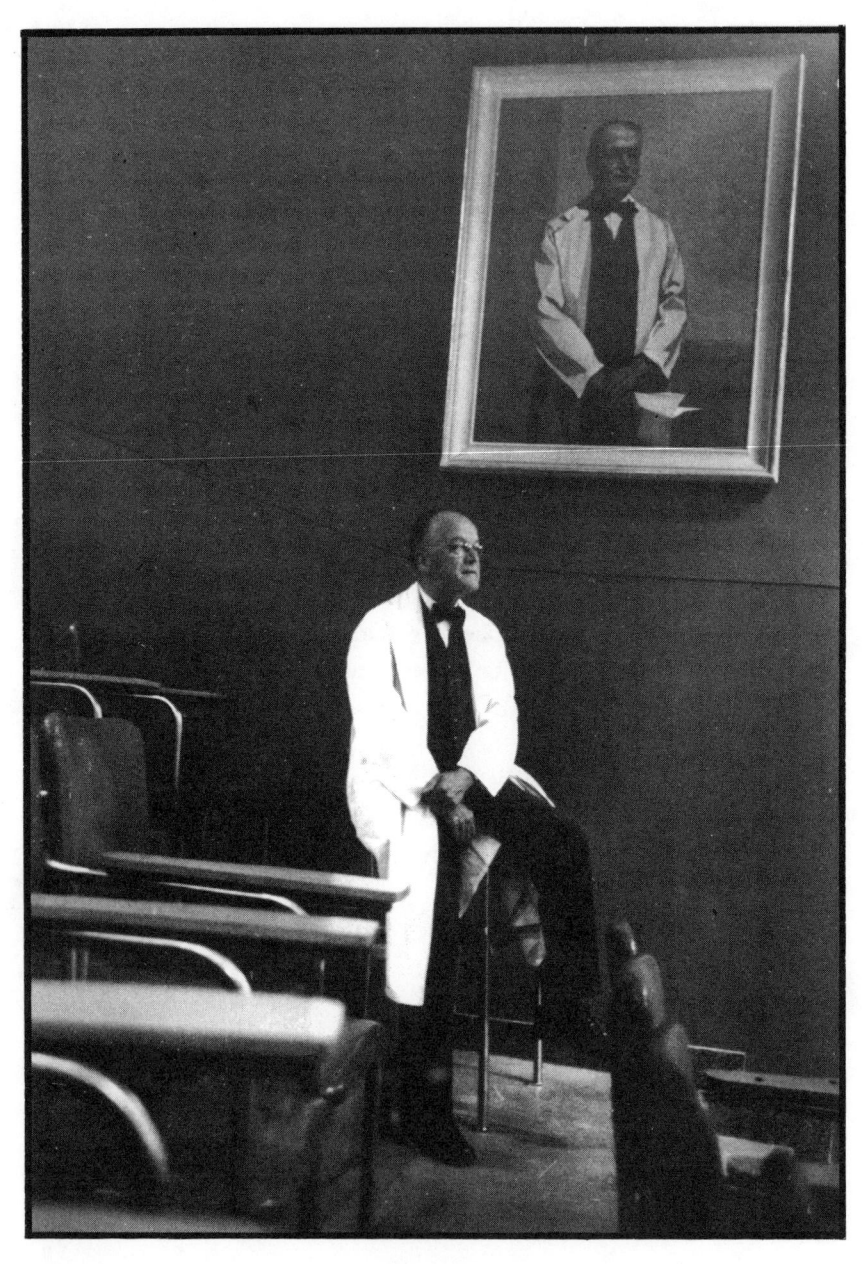

Alan Brown and the Cleeve Horne portrait in new lecture hall, 1951 (photo H.W. Tetlow, courtesy Maclean's Magazine*)*

Notes

Chapter 1

1. Royal Canadian Air Force
2. Prisoners of War
3. Dr. W.G. Scrimgeour, Parkhill, Ontario
4. Dr. C.P. Rance, Toronto
5. Internist on TGH (Toronto General Hospital) staff
6. Neurosurgeon on TGH staff
7. Dr. R.G.G. Allman, Brampton, Ontario
8. Dr. D.R. Clark, Peterborough, Ontario
9. Dr. J.B.J. McKendry, ed., *The Hospital for Sick Children: Dr. Alan Brown*, University of Toronto Press for HSC Alumni Association, 1984, p.34
10. Dr. D.R. Clark, Peterborough, Ontario

Chapter 2

1. Movie: *Hobson's Choice*, 1954, with Charles Laughton, directed by David Lean.
2. Sale, Charles (Chic), *The Specialist* (Toronto: McClelland and Stewart Limited, 1930).
3. Robert Mills, head of the Children's Aid Society.

Chapter 3

1. Dr. A. Lawrence Chute

2. ibid.
3. Alton Goldbloom, *Small Patients: The Autobiography of a Children's Doctor* (Toronto, 1959) p.135
4. Related by Elisabeth Fisher Lawson
5. Related by Barbara Alan Brown Kelley

Chapter 4

1. Rita Bristol Foster
2. McKendry, J.B.J. and J.D. Bailey, eds., *Paediatrics in Canada* (Ottawa: Canadian Paediatric Society, 1990) pp. 4-6
3. Drs. A.L. Chute and Nelles Silverthorne.
4. Dr. Nelles Silverthorne quoting Dr. Allen Baines
5. ibid.
6. As related by Barbara Alan Brown Kelley
7. Dr. A.L. Chute
8. Dr. Robert Farber
9. See Kerr, Robert B., and Douglas Waugh, *Duncan Graham, Medical Reformer and Educator* (Toronto: Dundurn Press Ltd., 1988)
10. ibid.
11. Dr. A.L. Chute

Chapter 5

1. Shelagh Hewitt Kareda, ed., "For Alison, and the World, 1918 was a Truly Momentous Year," *University College Alumni Magazine* (Fall 1992): 10-11
2. Grace Haldenby and Ruth Haldenby Mulholland
3. 1921 Boyd and Tisdall appointed Clinical Assistants. Boyd begins treatment of children with Banting and Best's newly discovered insulin.
4. Drs. A.D. Blackader (first president), Alan Brown, George Campbell, Crossan Clark, H.B. Cushing, Alton Goldbloom, D.B. Leitch and A.H. Spohn were the founders of the society.
5. Helen N. McCallum, RN
6. Phyllis Norton, RN
7. Hilda Rolstin, *The Hospital for Sick Children School of Nursing* (Toronto: HSC School of Nursing Alumnae Association, 1972), p.24
8. The HSC Medical Advisory Board minutes, 17/12/37 passed the recommendation that a letter be sent to the HSC Board of Trustees regarding the problem of insects in the hospital.

9. Dr. W.A. Hawke
10. HSC Medical Advisory Board minutes, 8/1/36
11. Dr. Helen Reid (Mrs. A. Lawrence Chute)
12. Dr. Frances Mulligan (Mrs. Donald H. McKay)
13. Nina Drake, technological staff member in HSC Nutritional Research Laboratories, directed by Dr. T.G.H. Drake. For a variant of this anecdote see also Marilyn Dunlop, *Bill Mustard* (Toronto, Dundurn Press, 1989), p. 16.
14. Dr. Eric C.H. Lehmann for Daffydil Night, 1944.
15. Dr. Bogoch, now practising in the U.S.A.
16. Dr. Walter F. Prendergast
17. Dr. Lillian Sugarman Clark
18. Dr. Howard (Pete) McGarrie
19. Dr. Helen Reid
20. ibid
21. Heather MacDougall, *Activists and Advocates: Toronto's Health Department 1883-1993* (Toronto, Dundurn Press, 1990) See also Donald Jones, "Historical Toronto: The man who made Toronto World's Healthiest City," *Toronto Daily Star* [Toronto] October 6,1990, p. M4.
22. Margaret D. Neilson, RN
23. Dr. Robert Farber
24. The proprietary name, Pablum, is a corruption of the Latin *pabulum* (food, nourishment)
25. Dr. Nelles Silverthorne
26. On January 10, 1945, Dr. Silverthorne assisted by Dr. Sugarman Clark administered penicillin to Bobby Van der Mullen who had a temperature of 107 degrees.
27. Miss Grace Haldenby
28. Helen N. McCallum, RN
29. Phyllis Norton, RN
30. Brown added to his prestige by attending the world-famous babies whose progress was followed in every detail by the daily press.
31. Phyllis Norton, RN
32. Margaret D. Neilson, RN
33. W.A. Hawke
34. Helen N. McCallum, RN
35. Dr. Bernard Laski paraphrasing Manace's letter
36. Royal assent to the Dionne Quintuplets Guardianship Act was signed

on 27 March 1935 by the Lieutenant-Governor of Ontario, the Hon. Herbert A. Bruce, himself a distinguished doctor.
37. Drs. A. Lawrence Chute and Helen Reid
38. Dr. Helen Reid
39. Dr. J.A. Peter Turner
40. Frederick Weinberg, "Dr. Alan Brown, Master Teacher," *Canadian Jewish News* (Toronto, 1975): 3-4.
41. A.I. Willinsky, *Memoirs*, (Toronto, 1960)
42. Dr. J.J. Slavens
43. Dr. Lillian Sugarman Clark
44. Margaret D. Neilson, RN
45. Mary Tisdall (Mrs. F.F. Tisdall)
46. Dr. J. Harry Ebbs
47. There is no trace of this paper
48. Nina Drake (Mrs. T.G.H. Drake)
49. This inscribed volume is in the Fisher Rare Book Room at the University of Toronto
50. Drs. Boyd, Chute, Donohue, Drake, Griffins, Hawke, Laski, McNaughton, Rance, E.C. Robertson, J. Ross, Snelling and Tisdall

Chapter 6

1. Bunt Smith Walker
2. Grace Haldenby
3. Dr. Nelles Silverthorne
4. Grace Haldenby
5. *Toronto Daily Star*, Saturday, August 6, 1932, p. 22
6. Lyn Carey Evans MacMillan
7. Grace Haldenby
8. Elisabeth Fisher Lawson
9. Dr. J.A. Peter Turner
10. Dr. W.A. Hawke
11. Brian Schwartz, "Fifth Column", *Globe and Mail* (Toronto), September 29, 1992, p. A24

Chapter 7

1. Elisabeth Fisher Lawson
2. William Woods, President, Gordon Mackay Knitting Mills
3. Barbara Alan Brown Kelley

4. Please see Chapter 2, note 2.
5. Mrs. F.N.G. Starr
6. Nancy Alan Brown Mayer
7. Women's Royal Canadian Naval Service (WRCNS), known as Wrens

Chapter 8

1. Dr. Nelles Silverthorne
2. Dr. M. Justin O'Brien
3. Grace Haldenby
4. Dr. A. Lawrence Chute
5. Deposited in HSC Archives
6. Dr. William A. Hawke
7. Dr. Frederick Weinberg
8. *Globe and Mail* (Toronto) 16 October 1954
9. Dr. Bernard Laski
10. Nancy Alan Brown Mayer
11. *The Hospital for Sick Children Annual Report 1960* (Toronto) p. 7
12. Now displayed between two other stained glass panels in the new chapel in the Atrium
13. Elisabeth Fisher Lawson

Appendix 1
A Selected List of Alan Brown's Publications

Books:
Brown, Alan, *The Normal Child. Its Care and Feeding* (Toronto: F.D. Goodchild, 1923) and (Toronto: McClelland & Stewart, 1926, 1932)
Brown, Alan & Frederick F. Tisdall, *Common Procedures in The Practice of Paediatrics* (Toronto: McClelland & Stewart, 1926, 1932, 1939)
Brown, Alan & George Campbell, *Infant Mortality*, [n.p] 1914

Unpublished:
Brown, Alan, *Nutrition of Infants*, [n.d.] part manuscript and part typescript, 2 vols., in The Hospital for Sick Children's Library.

Articles: Edited (with additions and corrections) from an abridged list* prepared somewhat haphazardly by Alan Brown for the 1943 questionnaire sent by the Toronto Academy of Medicine to all its members.

Often he simply added his name (following the custom of that day) to the hundreds of articles his HSC staff published. It is not now possible to distinguish with certainty between the articles in which his contribution was significant and those on which his name is listed as a co-author simply because of his position in the hospital. Therefore, unless he is

---

* In the library of the Toronto Academy of Medicine now housed in the Toronto General Division of the Toronto Hospital.

named as the sole or first author only those articles which research suggests were of particular interest to him have been listed. In addition, his list of publications has been arbitrarily reduced after 1933.

Brown, Alan, The luetin reaction in infancy. *Am. J. Dis. Child.* 6: 171-173, 1913

Holt, L. Emmett and Alan Brown, Results with salvarsan in hereditary syphilis. *Am. J. Dis. Child.* 6: 174-186, 1913

Chappell, W.F. and Alan Brown, Respiratory infections in infants' wards. *Am. J. Dis. Child.* 7: 380-382, 1914

Brown, Alan and Almon Fletcher, The Etiology of tetany — metabolic and clinical studies. *Am. J. Dis. Child.* 10: 313-30, 1915

Robertson, L. Bruce and Alan Brown, Blood transfusion in infants and young children. *Can. Med. Assoc. J.* 5: 298-305, 1915

Brown, Alan, Influenza meningitis with report of two cases. *Can. Med. Assoc. J.* 5: 1076-1080, 1915

Brown, Alan, Blood transfusion in haemorrhage of the newborn. *Can. Med. Assoc. J.* 6: 716-723, 1916

Brown, Alan, The ability of mothers to nurse their infants. *Can. Med. Assoc. J.* 7: 241-249, 1917

Brown, Alan, Duodenal ulcers in infancy. *Can. Med. Assoc. J.* 7: 320-323, 1917

Brown, Alan, Deficiency diseases of infancy and childhood. *Can. Med. Assoc. J.* 7: 911-924, 1917

Brown, Alan and G.E. Smith, The use of the longitudinal sinus for diagnostic and therapeutic measures in infancy. *Am. J. Dis. Child.* 13: 501-505, 1917

Brown, Alan and R. George, The care and feeding of the premature infant. *Archives of Pediatrics* 34: 609-616, 1917

Brown, Alan, H. Spohn and Ida F. Maclachlan, Protein milk. *Can. Med. Assoc. J.* 8: 510-522, 1918

Brown, Alan, Infant and child welfare work. *Public Health Journal* 9: 145-156, 1918

Brown, Alan, Problems of the rural mother in the feeding of her children. *Public Health Journal* 9: 297-301, 1918

Brown, Alan, G.E. Smith and G. Phillips, Auto-serum treatment of chorea. *Can. Med. Assoc. J.* 9: 52-62, 1919

Brown, Alan, Relation of the pediatrician to the community. *Public Health Journal* 10: 49-55, 1919

Brown, Alan and Ida F. MacLachlan, Protein milk powder. *Can. Med. Assoc. J.* 9: 528-537, 1919

*Brown, Alan, Child hygiene bureau. *California State Journal of Medicine* 17: 42ff, 1919

Brown, Alan, Toronto as a pediatric centre. *Canadian Medical Monthly* 5: 204-210, 1920

Brown, Alan, Ida F. MacLachlan and Roy Simpson, Effect of intravenous injections of calcium in tetany and the influence of cod liver oil and phosphorus in retention of calcium in the blood. *Am. J. Dis. Child* 19: 413-428, 1920

Brown, Alan, Factors to be considered in the construction of child's diet. *Can. Med. Monthly* 5: 398-406, 1920

Brown, Alan, Child Health. *Public Health Journal* 11: 49-53, 1920

Brown, Alan, Angelia M. Courtney and Ida F. MacLachlan, A clinical and metabolic study of acrodynia. *Archives of Pediatrics* 38: 609-628, 1921

Brown, Alan and G. Albert Davis, The prevalence of malnutrition in the public school children of Toronto. *Can. Med. Assoc. J.* 11: 124-126, 1921

Robertson, L. Bruce, Alan Brown and Roy Simpson, Blood transfusion in children, its indications and limitations. From an analysis of 600 cases. *Northwest Medicine* 20: 233-246, 1921

Brown, Alan, Ida F. MacLachlan and Roy Simpson, Cod-liver Oil without phosphorous as effective as cod-liver oil with phosphorous in rickets and tetany. *Can. Med. Assoc. J.* 11: 552-558, 1921

Brown, Alan, Angelia M. Courtney, F.F. Tisdall and Ida F. MacLachlan, A critical study of two cases of rickets developing in breast fed infants. *Archives of Pediatrics* 39: 559-66, 1922

Brown, Alan, Asthma in children. *Can. Med. Assoc. J.* 12: 780-786, 1922

Brown, Alan, Angelia M. Courtney and Ida F. MacLachlan, A clinical and chemical study of butter soup feeding in infants. *Am. J. Dis. Child.* 24: 368-81, 1922

Brown, Alan, Angelia M. Courtney and Ida F. MacLachlan, The effect of special high protein diets in the treatment of chronic intestinal indigestion in children. *British Journal of Children's Diseases* 19: 113-128, 1922

---

* Asterisks within list indicate articles were not seen by the author for checking.

Brown, Alan and Gladys Boyd, Acute Intestinal Intoxication in infants. An analysis of 75 cases treated in the HSC Toronto during the summer of 1922. *Can. Med. Assoc. J.* 13: 800-803, 1923

Brown, Alan, Treatment and general management of eczema in infants in private practice. *Can. Med. Assoc. J.* 13: 883-886, 1923

Brown, Alan, Certain features of child welfare not sufficiently emphasized. *Public Health Journal* 14: 243-249, 1923

*Brown, Alan, The treatment of septicaemias and intoxications in infants and children. *Wis. Med. J.* 23: 1924

Gallie, W.E. and Alan Brown, Acute haemorrhagic pancreatitis resulting from roundworms. *Am. J. Dis. Child.* 27: 192-194, 1924

*Brown, Alan and F.F. Tisdall, Factors involved in the acidity of stools of infants. *New York State Journal of Medicine* 25: 152-159, 1925

Brown, Alan, Angelia M. Courtney, G.A. Davis and Ida F. MacLachlan, Etiology of chronic intestinal indigestion. *Am. J. Dis. Child.* 30: 603-631, 1925.

Tisdall, F.F., T.G.H. Drake and Alan Brown, Carbohydrate metabolism of infants with diarrhea, infections and acute intestinal intoxication with a note on insulin. *Am. J. Dis. Child.* 30: 837-843, 1925

*Brown, Alan, The teaching of paediatrics in Canadian universities. *Transactions. 4th annual meeting, Canadian Society for the Study of Diseases of Children*: 1926

Brown, Alan, The role of The Hospital for Sick Children in correlating the agencies interested in child health. *Hospital Social Service* 16: 509-514, 1927

Morgan, E.A., A.H. Rolph and Alan Brown, Clinical manifestations of an enlarged thymus. *JAMA* 88: 703-706, 1927

Tisdall, F.F. and Alan Brown, Seasonal variation of the antirachitic effect of sunshine. *Am. J. Dis. Child.* 34: 721-736, 1927

Tisdall, F.F. and Alan Brown, Antirachitic effect of skyshine. *Am. J. Dis. Child.* 34: 737-741, 1927

Brown, Alan and F.F. Tisdall, Address on the seasonal variation of the antirachitic effect of sunshine and its effect on resistance to disease. *Can. Med. Assoc. J.* 17: 1425-1429, 1927.

Courtney, Angelia M. and Alan Brown, A comparison of the buffer capacity of various milk mixtures used in infant feeding. *Can. Med. Assoc. J.* 19: 52-55, 1928

Brown, Alan, Some common mistakes in diagnosis and therapy of diseases of children. *Can. Med. Assoc. J.* 19: 313-318, 1928

Brown, Alan, Sunlight — its effect on the growth of children and resistance to disease. *Canadian Public Health Journal* 29: 401-409, 1928

Brown, Alan and Angelia M. Courtney, The effect of digestion and assimilation of [fruit?] including bananas in the mixed diet of some children over five years of age. *Can. Med. Assoc. J.* 21: 37-42, 1929 [Word or words missing from the title as printed in journal]

Tisdall, F.F. and Alan Brown, The age, sex and seasonal incidence of certain diseases in children. *Am. J. Dis. Child.* 39: 163-173, 1930

Tisdall, F.F., Alan Brown, D.E.S. Wishart, T.G.H. Drake and M.M Johnson, Etiology of acute intestinal intoxication of infants: preliminary report. *South. Med. J.* 23: 107-112, 1930

Tisdall, F. F., T.G.H. Drake, Pearl Summerfeldt and Alan Brown, A new whole wheat irradiated biscuit containing vitamins and mineral elements. *Can. Med. Assoc. J.* 22: 166-170, 1930

Johnston, Marion M., Alan Brown and F.F. Tisdall, Enteral infections in acute intestinal intoxication. *Can. Med. Assoc. J.* 23: 231-237, 1930

Tisdall, F.F., T.G.H. Drake and Alan Brown, A new cereal mixture containing vitamins and mineral elements. *Am. J. Dis. Child.* 40: 791-799, 1930

Johnston, Marion M. and Alan Brown, Cases of intestinal intoxication in children attributed to B. dysenteriae sonne. *Can. Med. Assoc. J.* 24: 364-372, 1931

Brown, Alan, Preventive pediatrics and its relation to the general practitioner. *Can. Med. Assoc. J.* 24: 517-522, 1931

Tisdall, F.F., T.G.H. Drake and Alan Brown, The incorporation of vitamins in bread. *Can. Med. Assoc. J.* 24: 210-213, 1931.

Summerfeldt, Pearl, T.G.H. Drake and Alan Brown. The treatment of acute intestinal intoxication. *Can. Med. Assoc. J.* 25: 288-292, 1931

Summerfeldt, Pearl, F.F. Tisdall and Alan Brown, The curative effects of cereals and biscuits on experimental anaemias. *Can. Med. Assoc. J.* 26: 666-669, 1932

Johnston, Marion M., Alan Brown, F.F. Tisdall and Donald T. Fraser, Intestinal infections in infants. *Am. J. Dis. Child.* 45: 1-17, 1933

Johnston, Marion M., Alan Brown and Mildred J. Kaake, Intestinal infection in infants and children, 1930 and 1931 series. *Am. J. Dis. Child.* 45: 498-505, 1933

Brown, Alan and Nelles Silverthorne, Meningococcic meningitis in infancy: report of case. *JAMA* 101: 272-273, 1933

Brown, Alan and F.F. Tisdall, The role of minerals and vitamins in growth and resistance to infection. *British Medical Journal* 1: 55-57, 1933. Read at the British Medical Assocation Centenary Meeting London, January 14, 1932.

Brown, Alan, Acute intestinal intoxication. *Canadian Public Health Journal* 24: 57-64, 1933

Brown, Alan, The prevention of neonatal mortality. *Can. Med. Assoc. J.* 29: 264-268, 1933

Brown, Alan and F.F. Tisdall, Effect of vitamins and inorganic elements on growth and resistance to disease in children. *Annals of Internal Medicine* 7: 342-352, 1933

*Brown, Alan, Some common errors in the diagnosis and treatment of children. *Mississippi Doctor*, 1934

Snelling, C.E., and Alan Brown, A clinical application of haematology to infants and children. *Can. Med. Assoc. J.* 30: 488-494, 1934

*Brown, Alan, Feeding of the newborn. *Medical Press* and *Circular cxci*, no. 5033: 1935

Brown, Alan, Appendiceal colic. *Can. Med. Assoc. J.* 38: 445-455, 1938

Brown, Alan, The value of pasteurization. *Canadian Public Health Journal* 29: 318-320, 1938

Brown, Alan, Some factors concerning the care of the newborn. *Canadian Public Health Journal* 29: 337-344, 1938

Brown, Alan, Child care during war. *Can. Med. Assoc. J.* 42: 257-260, 1940

Brown, Alan, How the children's hospital can best meet community needs. *Hospitals*: 42-45, 1940. Read at the 41st convention of the American Hospitals Association, Toronto, 25-29 Sept.1939.

*Brown, Alan, Abdominal pediatric conditions. *Tex. Med.* 36: 482ff., 1940

Brown, Alan. A decade of paediatric progress. Read at the fourth Blackader lecture 19 June 1940. *Can. Med. Assoc. J.* 43: 305-313, 1940

*Brown, Alan. A consideration of some common pediatric problems. *Tex. Med.* 36: 778ff, 1941

Brown, Alan and Elizabeth C. Robertson. Essential features concerning the proper nutrition of the infant and child. *Can. Med. Assoc. J.* 48: 297-302, 1943

*Brown, Alan. 1948. Gave the Engleby lectures at Queen's College, Birmingham, England.

Brown, Alan. The Frederick F. Tisdall Memorial Lecture. *Can. Med. Assoc. J.* 64: 263-265, 1951. Read at the annual meeting of the Society for the Diseases of Children, Niagara Falls, Ontario, 1950.

Brown, Alan. Paediatrics: Recent advances of interest to the general practitioners. *University of Western Ontario Medical Journal* 22: 135-146, 1952. Given at the Eccles Memorial Lectureship 2 June 1950.

Brown, Alan, Paediatrics: Recent advances of interest to the general practitioners. [Conclusion]. *University of Western Ontario Medical Journal* 23: 33-49, 1953. Given at the Eccles Memorial Lectureship 1 October 1952.

Appendix 2

Some sources interviewed and quoted

Boddington, Dr. George D.M., graduated from University of Toronto 1937, anaesthetist at Toronto General Hospital. Semi-retired.

Bruce-Robertson, Dr. Alan, Class of '50, Alan Brown's namesake, son of Dr. Bruce Robertson. Research Associate at the University of Toronto.

Chute, Dr. A. Lawrence, HSC paediatrician 1937, PhD in physiology 1939. HSC's Physician-in-Chief 1951-1966. Dean of Medicine, University of Toronto 1966-1976. Married to Dr. Helen Reid. Retired.

Clark, Dr. Donald R., Alan Brown's chief resident 1948-9 during the "locked door" episode. Currently practising paediatrics in Peterborough, Ontario.

Clark, Dr. Lillian M. Sugarman, chief resident 1943-5. Practised in paediatric clinic, Niagara Falls, Ontario. Recently retired.

Drake, Nina, from 1929 research assistant to Dr. T.G.H. Drake who succeeded Dr. F.F. Tisdall as Director HSC Research Laboratories. Retired 1952.

Ebbs, Adele Statten, former director Camp Wapomeo, married to Dr. J. Harry Ebbs, first full-time salaried HSC staff member 1946.

Farber, Dr. Robert, HSC staff since 1952. Senior intern, "locked door" episode. 1955-8 took Alan Brown's house calls and summer office.

Haldenby, Grace, Alan Brown's private practice secretary 1927-58. Ruth Haldenby Mulholland added further details to her sister's tales of the many years she worked for Alan Brown.

Hawke, Dr. W.A., Alan Brown's chief resident 1933-4, HSC staff in neuropsychiatry and paediatrics since 1935. Emeritus Professor (Paediatrics), University of Toronto.

Kelley, Barbara Alan Brown, a great admirer of her father. A source of many anecdotes of family life at home and at their summer cabin, Sequoia.

Laski, Dr. Bernard, paediatrician and pathologist on HSC staff since 1948. Emeritus Professor (Paediatrics), University of Toronto.

Lawson, Elizabeth Fisher, Alan Brown's niece. Her anecdotes and comments describe the early years of the Browns' domestic life.

Lehmann, Dr. Eric C. H., University of Toronto, Class of '45. Head of orthopaedics at St. Paul's Hospital, Vancouver. Retired.

McCallum, Helen N., RN, 1930-37 Montreal Children's Hospital. 1939 appointed first full-time clinical instructor student nurses HSC. Retired.

MacDonald, Dr. Keith, University of Toronto Class of '45. Toronto General Hospital ophthalmologist since 1947. Semi-retired.

McGarry, Dr. Howard (Pete), Alan Brown's chief resident 1934-5. Senior paediatrician, Niagara Falls, Ontario.

McKay, Dr. Frances Mulligan, Alan Brown's first female chief resident, January 1938; resigned in May to marry Dr. Donald H. McKay.

MacMillan, Eluned Carey Evans, environmentalist, granddaughter of David Lloyd George, married to Dr. Robert L. MacMillan.

MacMillan, Dr. Robert L., Toronto General Hospital staff since 1945, co-developer of monitored cardiac intensive care unit now used worldwide. Emeritus Professor (Internal Medicine), University of Toronto.

Mayer, Nancy Alan Brown, younger daughter of Alan Brown whom she admired and loved but could not easily reach.

Neilson, Margaret D., RN, HSC staff 1935-1953. Instructor on infant wards and Alan Brown's clinic nurse. Retired.

Norton, Phyllis, RN, won Operating Room scholarship, HSC staff 1936-78, head nurse, ear, nose and throat operating room. Retired.

O'Brien, Dr. M. Justin (Gus), HSC surgical intern, three years chief resident St. Michael's Hospital, Alan Brown's chief resident 1950-51 then HSC staff. Semi-retired.

Prendergast, Dr. Walter F., Class of '50. General practitioner and physician to the T. Eaton Company. Semi-retired.

Rance, Dr. C. P., Alan Brown's chief resident 1949-50 during the "locked door" caper, then HSC staff. Retired.

Dr. Helen Reid, HSC intern 1939, paediatrician at Infants' Home, author and editor. 1951 organized HSC Women's Auxiliary. Married to Dr. A.L. Chute. Retired.

Ross, Dr. Colin S., Class of '50. Vice-President and Medical Director of Munich Re-insurance Company of Canada. Retired.

Silverthorne, Dr. Nelles, Alan Brown's chief resident 1929-30. Developed whooping cough vaccine from live viral cultures. HSC Honorary Consultant.

Slavens, Dr. John J., graduated 1930, postgraduate studies New York, and three-year fellowship Mayo Clinic. HSC staff 1944 -1970. Died 1993.

Tisdall, Mary, wife of Dr. Frederick F. Tisdall, Director, HSC Research Laboratories. Mary died in 1994, Frederick died in 1949.

Turner, Dr. J.A. Peter, HSC staff since 1948. Currently senior consultant HSC and Professor Emeritus, Department of Paediatrics, U. of T.

Weinberg, Dr. Fred, HSC staff since 1950, on call for Alan Brown 1951-1954. Associate Director HSC Child Development Clinic 1973-91.

Appendix 3

Books and theses consulted

Berton, Pierre. *The Dionne Years* (Toronto: McClelland & Stewart, 1977)
Braithwaite, Max. *Sick Kids: The Story of The Hospital for Sick Children in Toronto* (Toronto: McClelland & Stewart, 1974)
Gilday, Diane. "The Founding and the First Quarter Century of Management of The Hospital for Sick Children" (University of Toronto MA thesis, 1991)
Goldbloom, Alton. *Small Patients: The Autobiography of a Children's Doctor* (Toronto: Longmans, 1959)
McKendry, J.B.J., co-ordinator. *Dr. Alan Brown* (Hospital for Sick Children Alumni Association and University of Toronto Press, 1984)
McKendry, J.B.J., and J.D. Bailey. *Paediatrics in Canada* (Ottawa: Canadian Paediatric Society and Conestoga Press, 1990)
McRae, Sandra F. "The 'Scientific Spirit' in Medicine at the University of Toronto, 1880-1910" (Univ. of Toronto PhD thesis, 1987)
Rolstin, Hilda. *The History of the Hospital for Sick Children School of Nursing* (Toronto: HSC School of Nursing Alumnae Association, 1972)

Index

Ahmic Lake, 91, 123, 144, 150, 183, 185, 197
Allman, R.G.G., 14, 15
"Annie and Norah" (A.B.'s domestic staff), 135, 155, 165
anti-Semitism, 94 ff
Austin, Pearl, 58

Baines, Allen, 50, 51, 52
Baker, E., 195
Balmforth, Harry, 90
Barnett, H.J.M., 194
Bell, Whiteford, 42
Best, Charles, 66
Blackader, A.D., 47
Boddington, George D.M., 194
Bogoch, Dr., 63
Bower, Joseph, 61, 79, 84, 90, 177
Boxhill, Miss, 78
Boyd, Gladys, 57
Brown, Alan (blackballed by American Pediatric Society), 103
— Daffydil Night, 63
— funeral, 195
— good hygiene, 64, 65
— honeymoon in Germany, 43, 44
— hospital appointments, 91
— internships, 38
— Jarvis Collegiate, 26
— move to new hospital, 172
— Model School, 25
— Physician-in-Chief, 57
— plagiarism, 103 ff
— professor of new department of paediatrics, 53
— residency at Babies' Hospital NYC, 39
— return to Canada, 46
— Silver Medal, 21
— stroke, 190 ff
— U of T Athletic Association, 33
Brown, Barbara (Barbara Alan Brown Kelley), 22, 26, 78, 128, 131, 145, 155, 159, 183, 190
Brown, Clinton, 19, 25, 42
Brown, Connie (see also Constance Hobbs), 38, 39, 107, 121, 157 ff, 190
— Needlework Guild, 94

Brown, Donald, 19, 25, 42
Brown, George, 21, 22
Brown, Margery, 19, 25, 42
Brown, Nancy, 131, 184 ff, 197
Bruce, Herbert, 89, 116
Bruce-Robertson, Alan, 14, 15, 56

Canadian Paediatric Society, 58
Cassidy, Mary, 121, 165
Chisholm, Juliet, 94
Chute, L.A., 12, 66, 73, 91, 119, 125, 177, 178, 194
Clark, D.R., 15
Clark, Lillian Sugarman, 85, 94, 97
Courtney, Angelia, 67, 69, 104
Czerny, Adalbert, 41

Daffydil Night, 63
Dafoe, Allan, 88
Dampsey, Jack, 165
Davey, Jean, 94
Diamond, Mrs., 122
Dionne quintuplets, 88
Drake, Nina, 176, 192
Drake, T.G.H., 67 ff, 82, 102, 105

Eaton, Lady, 116 ff
Eaton's, College Street stables, 61
Ebbs, Harry, 49, 94, 102, 148, 177
Edwards, Hal, 81, 83
Edwards, Florence, 81
Eiweissmilch, 41

Farber, R., 16, 85, 126, 177, 178, 180, 186
Finkelstein, Heinrich, 41, 42
Fisher, Grant, 156, 162, 197
Fisher, Tot, 131, 162, 163
Fletcher, Jack, 83
Flexner, Abraham, 149
Fortier, René, 47
Fraser, Donald, 63
Frost, Premier Leslie, 195

Gallie, Gordon, 35, 63, 181
Gallie, W. Edward, 49, 63, 95
George, Ruggles, 42
George, (A.B.'s Chinese cook), 134
Goldbloom, Alton, 47, 81, 95

Goodchild, S., 81, 123
Gooderham, Steve, 163
Gowans, Annie, 22
Gowans, Gavina, 21
Gowans, Grace, 21
Gowans, Susan, 21
Graham, Duncan, 52, 63
Graham, Enid, 53
Graham, Roscoe, 63
Greenwood, W.F., 184
Grier, Stella, 123
Groves, Mrs., 69
Guggenheim brothers, 40

Haldenby, Doris, 109, 185, 191
Haldenby, Grace, 107 ff, 122, 123, 185 ff, 193
Haldenby, Ruth (Mulholland), 109, 114
Haney, Eva, 42
Hastings, Charles, 66
Hawke, William A., 73 ff, 82, 91, 126
Hepburn, Mitchell, 66, 89 ff
Hobbs, Anne Osborne, 33
Hobbs, Constance (see also Brown, Connie), 33, 42
Hobbs, Mr. and Mrs. Richard, 26, 33
Hobbs, Sarah, 33
Hobbs, Yvonne, 42
Hogg, Bill, 14
Holt, Emmett, 39, 41, 79
Horne, Cleeve, 176, 197
Hospitals:
  Babies' Hospital, New York, 67, 79
  Children's Hospital of Eastern Ontario, 83
  Children's Hospital, Halifax, 47
  Children's Hospital, Winnipeg, 47
  Children's Memorial Hospital, Montreal, 47
  convalescent hospital, Thistletown, 80
  Homewood Health Centre, 187 ff
  Infants' Home, 125
  L'Hôpital Ste. Justine pour les Enfants, Montreal, 47
  Scarborough General Hospital, 83
Hospital for Sick Children:
  College Street building, 59
  dress code, 58
  infant mortality, 50, 52
  new building on University Avenue, 64
  nursing staff, 58
  nutritional laboratories, 57, 67, 68
  Research Institute, 69
Hurricane Hazel, 185
Hurst Brown, Dr., 113

influenza epidemic, 55 ff
iron lung, 90

Jackson, Joseph, 82
Jacobi, Abraham, 39 ff, 183
Johnson, R.H., 178
Johnson, Ross, 193

Kane, Josephine, 62
Karger, Dr., 94
Kelley, Ann, 43, 44
Kelley, Bill, 156
Kelley, Tim, 68, 197
Keith, John, 81
Keith, W. S., 76
Kirkpatrick, Peggy, 125

Laidlaw, Robert A., 80, 173, 195
Laski, Bernard, 72, 81, 178, 180
Lawson, Elisabeth Fisher, 33, 107, 131, 132, 156, 163
Leverings, the, 198

Macdonald, Sir John A., 21
Machell, H. T., 106
Mackenzie, W. L., rebellion, 20
MacMillan, R. L., 12
Manace, Gordon, 83, 180
Massey, Raymond, 33
Masten, Jean, 58, 145
McCallum, Helen, 50, 99
McCormick, R. R. (*Chicago Tribune*), 131
McCreary, Dr., 80, 88
McCurdy, P., 132
McFarlane, Dean J., 12
McGarry, H., 19, 84
McKay, Donald, 61
McKenzie, K.G., 14
Meyer, L. F., 41
Mills, Robert, 26
Morgan, Edward (Ted), 42, 50, 163, 165, 180
Mulligan, Frances, 61
Mustard, W. T., 62, 76

Neilson, Margaret, D., 14, 89, 97, 100
Norton, Phyllis, 76, 176

O'Brien, Justin, 72, 176, 180
Oille, John, 85, 94, 137
Osborne, Sarah, 155

Pablum, 67 ff
Paediatric Research Foundation, 68
Panton, Kathleen, 58
Park, F., 83
pasteurization, 66, 89 ff

Peacock, Lady, 131
Phillips, Mayor Nathan, 195
poliomyelitis, 90
Prendergast, W. F., 15

Rafflaub, Thelma, 145, 183
Rance, C.P., 13, 14, 15
Rathbun, Marjorie, 42
Reichert, Harold, 14
Reid, Helen, 26, 61, 73, 119, 125
Rickard, Tessie, 109
Riel, L. rebellion, 20
Roaring Twenties, 56
Robertson, Bruce, 42, 50, 56
Robertson, D. Edward, 76, 95, 97, 116, 150, 163
Robertson, Donald, 159
Robertson, Elizabeth Chant, 104
Robertson, Enid, 53
Robertson, John Ross, 50, 51, 59, 172
Ross, Colin S., 13

Sass-Kortsak, S., 120
"Sequoia", 144, 198
Scrimgeour, W. G., 13
Shulman, Morton, 100
Shirley, Sen. Swager, 150
Silverthorne, N., 16, 49, 68, 80, 102, 117, 121, 124, 137, 149, 177, 180, 187, 193, 195
Simpson, Roy, 128
Slavens, Jack, 75, 83, 104, 124, 180
Smith, D. (Baron Strathcona & Mount Royal), 21
Smith, Mary Agnes, 39

Snelling, Peter, 81
Sparrow, Muriel, 116
Sparrow, Robert, 116
Spence, Sir James, 177
Starr, Mrs. F. N. G., 160
Strathy, George, 42
Strauss, Nathan, 40, 41
Sugarman, Lillian, 69
Sunwheat biscuits, 68
Sutherland, "Sudsy", 13

Tamblyn, Mrs., 122
Tilman, W. J., 47
Tisdall, Charles, 104
Tisdall, F. F., 67 ff, 102, 104, 149, 184
Tisdall, Mary, 104, 149
Toronto society, 25 ff
Turner, J. A. P., 13

Van Wyck, H. B., 63

Wansborough, T., 177
War, American Civil, 20
Warren, Helen, 42
Weech, Ashley, 104
Weinberg, Fred, 68, 76, 95, 180, 185
Weinberg, Sari, 65
Well Baby Clinics, 94
White, George, 183
William (A.B.'s chauffeur), 120, 128, 134
Willinsky, A. I., 95
Wishart, D. J. G., 76
Wood, I. W., 47
Woods, William, 145, 148

PRINTED IN CANADA